The Role of Companion Animals in the Treatment of Mental Disorders

The Role of Companion Animals in the Treatment of Mental Disorders

EDITED BY

Nancy R. Gee, Ph.D.
Lisa D. Townsend, Ph.D., LCSW
Robert L. Findling, M.D., M.B.A.

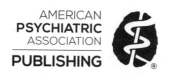

AMERICAN
PSYCHIATRIC
ASSOCIATION
PUBLISHING

If you wish to buy 50 or more copies of the same title, please go to www.appi.org/specialdiscounts for more information.

Copyright © 2023 American Psychiatric Association Publishing

ALL RIGHTS RESERVED

First Edition

Manufactured in the United States of America on acid-free paper
27 26 25 24 23   5 4 3 2 1

ISBN 978-1-61537-455-7 (paperback), 978-1-61537-456-4 (ebook)

American Psychiatric Association Publishing
800 Maine Avenue SW, Suite 900
Washington, DC 20024–2812
www.appi.org

Library of Congress Cataloging-in-Publication Data
A CIP record is available from the Library of Congress.

British Library Cataloguing in Publication Data
A CIP record is available from the British Library.

Contents

Contributors

Jessica Bibbo, Ph.D.
Research Scientist, Center for Research and Education, Benjamin Rose Institute on Aging, Cleveland, Ohio

Peter F. Buckley, M.D.
Chancellor, University of Tennessee Health Science Center, Memphis, Tennessee

Alexa M. Carr, Ph.D.
Lecturer, Department of Human Development, Washington State University, Pullman, Washington

Cynthia K. Chandler, Ed.D.
Professor, Department of Counseling and Higher Education, University of North Texas, Denton, Texas

Ann Childress, M.D.
President, Center for Psychiatry and Behavioral Medicine, Inc., Las Vegas, Nevada

Laura Dunn, M.D.
Chair, Department of Psychiatry; Director, Psychiatric Research Institute; and Marie Wilson Howells Professor, University of Arkansas for Medical Sciences, Little Rock, Arkansas

Robert L. Findling, M.D., M.B.A.
Professor and Chair, Department of Psychiatry, and C. Kenneth and Diane Wright Distinguished Chair in Clinical and Translational Research, Virginia Commonwealth University, Richmond, Virginia

Aubrey H. Fine, Ed.D.
Professor Emeritus, Licensed Psychologist, California Polytechnic State University, Pomona, California

Erika Friedmann, Ph.D.
Professor and Associate Dean for Research, University of Maryland School of Nursing, Baltimore, Maryland

Nancy R. Gee, Ph.D.
Professor, Department of Psychiatry; Director, Center for Human-Animal Interaction; and Bill Balaban Chair in Human-Animal Interaction, Virginia Commonwealth University School of Medicine, Richmond, Virginia

Sgt. David Hibler, M.S.
Ph.D. Student, Evolution Ecology and Organismal Biology, Ohio State University, Columbus, Ohio

Jennifer Hightower, Ph.D., NCC
Assistant Professor, Department of Counseling, ISU Meridian Sam and Aline Skaggs Health Science Center, Idaho State University, Meridian, Idaho

Abigail M. Jacaruso, OTD, OTR
Occupational Therapist, Dogwood Therapy Services, Albuquerque, New Mexico

Susan G. Kornstein, M.D.
Professor of Psychiatry and Executive Director, Institute for Women's Health, Virginia Commonwealth University, Richmond, Virginia

Cheryl A. Krause-Parello, Ph.D., R.N., FAAN
Associate Dean for Research and Scholarship, and Professor, Christine E. Lynn College of Nursing, Florida Atlantic University, Boca Raton, Florida

James Levenson, M.D.
Rhona Arenstein Professor of Psychiatry and Chair of the Division of Consultation/Liaison Psychiatry, Virginia Commonwealth University School of Medicine, Richmond, Virginia

Alice R. Mao, M.D.
Professor of Psychiatry and Behavioral Sciences, Baylor College of Medicine, Houston, Texas; and Director, Texas Children's Hospital, Child and Adolescent Psychiatry Autism and Developmental Disorders Clinic

Aubrey L. Milatz, M.S.
Doctoral Student, Department of Human Development, Washington State University, Pullman, Washington

S. Julianna Moreno, B.S.N.
Research Assistant, Christine E. Lynn College of Nursing, Florida Atlantic University, Boca Raton, Florida

Megan K. Mueller, Ph.D.
Associate Professor, Department of Clinical Sciences, Cummings School of Veterinary Medicine at Tufts University, N. Grafton, Massachusetts

Leanne O. Nieforth, Ph.D.
Postdoctoral Research Associate, College of Veterinary Medicine, University of Arizona, Tucson, Arizona

Marguerite E. O'Haire, Ph.D.
Professor, Associate Dean for Research, College of Veterinary Medicine, University of Arizona, Tucson, Arizona

Patricia Pendry, Ph.D.
Professor, Department of Human Development, Washington State University, Pullman, Washington

Beth A. Pratt, Ph.D., R.N.
Assistant Professor of Nursing, Christine E. Lynn College of Nursing, Florida Atlantic University, Boca Raton, Florida

Kerri E. Rodriguez, Ph.D.
Postdoctoral Research Fellow, Human-Animal Bond in Colorado, School of Social Work, Colorado State University, Fort Collins, Colorado

Sabrina E. B. Schuck, Ph.D.
Assistant Professor in Residence, Pediatrics, School of Medicine, University of California, Irvine, Irvine, California

Leslie Stewart, Ph.D., LCPC, C-AAIS
Associate Professor, Department of Counseling, Idaho State University, Pocatello, Idaho

Tushar P. Thakre, M.D., Ph.D.
Associate Professor and Chair, Division of Inpatient Psychiatry; and Medical Director, Inpatient/Acute Psychiatry and Neuromodulation Department of Psychiatry, Virginia Commonwealth University School of Medicine, Richmond, Virginia

Ayse Torres, Ph.D., LMHC, CRC
Assistant Professor, Clinical Rehabilitation Counseling, College of Education, Florida Atlantic University, Boca Raton, Florida

Lisa D. Townsend, Ph.D., LCSW
Associate Professor, Departments of Pediatrics and Psychiatry, Children's Hospital of Richmond; and Clinical and Research Associate, Center for Human-Animal Interaction, Virginia Commonwealth University, Richmond, Virginia

Jaymie L. Vandagriff, Ph.D.
Lecturer, Department of Human Development, Washington State University, Pullman, Washington

Melissa Y. Winkle, OTR/L, FAOTA, CPDT-KA
Owner, Occupational Therapist, and Professional Dog Trainer, Dogwood Therapy Services, Albuquerque, New Mexico

Disclosures

The following contributors to this book have indicated a financial interest in or other affiliation with a commercial supporter, a manufacturer of a commercial product, a provider of a commercial service, a nongovernmental organization, and/or a government agency, as listed below:

Ann Childress, M.D., has received research support from Allergan, Emalex Biosciences, Akili, Otsuka, Purdue Pharma, Adlon Therapeutics, and Supernus Pharmaceuticals. She has been a consultant for Lumos, Otsuka, Purdue Pharma, KemPharm, and Supernus Pharmaceuticals. She has served on an advisory board for Sunovion, Supernus Pharmaceuticals, and Noven. She has been a speaker for Takeda Pharmaceutical Company, Ironshore, Tris Pharma, Corium, and Supernus

Pharmaceuticals. She has received writing support from Takeda Pharmaceutical Company and Noven.

Robert L. Findling, M.D., M.B.A., has received research support, acted as a consultant, and received honoraria from Adamas Pharmaceuticals, Afecta Pharmaceuticals, Akili, Alkermes, American Academy of Child and Adolescent Psychiatry, American Psychiatric Association Publishing, Idorsia, Lundbeck, MJH Life Sciences, National Institutes of Health, Otsuka, PaxMedica, Patient-Centered Outcomes Research Institute, Pfizer, Physicians Postgraduate Press, Receptor Life Sciences, Signant Health, Sunovion, Supernus Pharmaceuticals, Syneos Health, Takeda Pharmaceutical Company, Teva Pharmaceutical Industries, Tris Pharma, and Viatris.

Nancy R. Gee, Ph.D., received a Mars Petcare unrestricted grant for research on loneliness in hospitalized patients (active – older adults), a Human Animal Bond Research Institute grant for research on loneliness in hospitalized patients (active – inpatient psychiatry), and a Nestle Purina grant for research on loneliness in hospitalized children (active).

Susan G. Kornstein, M.D., is a consultant for Lilly, AbbVie, Janssen, and Sage Therapeutics.

Sabrina E. B. Schuck, Ph.D., received Health & Human Development Award 103422, Grant 1289454.

Foreword

TIMMY WAS NEVER IN THE WELL.

Yet, the phrase "Lassie! Timmy's in the well," inspired by a 60-year-old television show, lives on. It has become a meme, passed on through generations, signifying the ability of nonhuman animals to rescue us from danger or, perhaps more accurately, our desire that they do so.

Many of us have felt rescued by a dog. We don't need to be trapped in a well to wonder if we would have made it through something—the pandemic, sexual abuse, profound grief—without a dog on our couch. However, enjoying the companionship of a strokable, sentient, emotionally receptive mammal does not tell us if dogs, or other animals, can be constructively involved in the therapeutic treatment of mental illness and developmental disorders.

This could be true for many reasons, perhaps best suggested, at its deepest level, by the words of John Muir: "I only went for a walk, and finally concluded to stay out till sundown, for going out, I found, was really going in." The fact is, as special as we humans might be—with our busy brains and our elaborate communication—we do not "just happen to inhabit" the world, as David Abram reminds us in *Becoming Animal: An Earthly Cosmology*.[1] Other animals (and the land around them) are "as much within us as they are around us" (p. 77).

Perhaps this is another way of saying that we all need to feel connected. Humans are highly social animals, but the need to be with others is not necessarily confined to members of the same species. Biologist Edward O. Wilson popularized the concept of *biophilia*,[2] "the urge to affiliate with other forms of life," while Richard Louv, in the *Last Child in the*

---

[1] Abram D: Becoming Animal: An Earthly Cosmology. New York, Vintage Books, 2011

[2] Wilson EO: Biophilia. Cambridge, MA, Harvard University Press, 1984

Woods: Saving Our Children From Nature-Deficit Disorder,[3] coined the phrase *nature-deficit disorder* to emphasize that to be truly healthy, people need to feel close to the natural world around them, including animals, plants, and the land. This is not news to the peoples of many cultures, including members of many Native American tribes, but has, until recently, been counter to the perspective of classic Western philosophy.

At a more proximal level, we know that nonhuman animals are often seen as givers of unconditional love and affection. In part, this is no doubt because they cannot use human language. I have joked in many a speech that it is a good thing that dogs can't talk, because we wouldn't always like what they have to say. Every animal behaviorist and dog trainer can tell you a story in which they would bet the farm that an animal's facial expression would translate into something unprintable. However, our perception of unconditional love is based on far more than a lack of language. As is described in detail in Chapter 1, "Introduction," and many of the chapters that follow, many adults and children have emotional attachments to companion animals on par with those of their siblings. Dogs, for one, can "get us coming and going," as I write in *For the Love of a Dog: Understanding Emotion in You and Your Best Friend.*[4] They can provide a sense of the unconditional love we all desire from our parents, while, because of their relative helplessness, eliciting feelings in us of parental love and nurturance.

These attachments are not one-directional. Social and highly emotional animals like dogs, horses, and, yes, cats clearly form strong attachments to their humans that are often equally powerful, driven by a shared mammalian physiology that shows, for example, an increase in oxytocin during relaxed gazes between dogs and their owners. Although oxytocin is a far more complicated hormone than is sometimes portrayed in the popular press, its deficits appear to be a potentially important player in many psychiatric challenges, including autism and anxiety disorders.

But is this enough to support the idea that animals can, or should, be involved in the treatment of mental illness or disability? Or to tell us which animals? For whom? In what way? Not at all, which is why the science presented in this book is so important. Decades ago, when I was

---

[3] Louv R: Last Child in the Woods: Saving our Children from Nature-Deficit Disorder, Revised and Updated Edition. Chapel Hill, NC, Algonquin Books of Chapel Hill, 2008

[4] McConnell PB: For the Love of a Dog: Understanding Emotion in You and Your Best Friend. New York, Ballantine Books, 2007

starting out as an applied animal behaviorist, the head pharmacist at the University of Wisconsin School of Veterinary Medicine told me that if a drug had the power to do good, then it had the power to do harm. That is also true of animal-assisted therapy (AAT) and animal-assisted interventions (AAIs).

I remember a client I had years ago, a middle-aged devoted mother with a 12-year-old son on the autism spectrum. She had adopted a dog for him, based on the recommendation of a professional, in the belief that the dog would provide companionship and, she was promised, an increase in the child's ability to communicate. By the time I came into the picture, the dog and the child were terrified of each other.

She wanted me to fix it. I couldn't begin to, unless you define fixing as explaining that the situation was untenable. The dog was a highly reactive and sensitive herding breed, who barked when he became aroused at fast, erratic movements. The child was overwhelmed by the dog's movements and barking and flapped his arms and screamed when they happened, which set off the dog, which set off the child. It was a heartbreaking cycle of dysfunction and suffering and an illustration of why it is vital that each case is carefully evaluated. After doing my best to explain that the situation was unfair to both her child and the dog, I was summarily dismissed. I never knew how it sorted out.

This is why the information contained in, for example, Chapter 7, "Companion Animals in the Treatment of Autism Spectrum Disorder," is so valuable. As in other chapters, the authors emphasize what factors lead to successful outcomes (or failures). They summarize the results of 85 studies, which suggest that AAI can lead to increased social interactions, along with improved communication abilities, in some cases, in some environments. However, as is often the case in this field, the authors also note concerns with methodology, small sample sizes, and a lack of randomized controlled trial designs.

The Centers for Disease Control and Prevention estimates that 1 in 25 Americans lives with a serious mental illness, and the National Institute of Mental Health stated that in 2020, 1 in 5 adults in the United States had "any mental illness." We are in desperate need of information about how to prevent and treat these debilitating conditions more effectively. Editors Gee, Townsend, and Findling have done prodigious work collecting state-of-the-art knowledge about when and how companion animals can be involved effectively in the treatment of mental illness and developmental disorders and the promotion of mental health.

The information in this book is a critical antidote to two of the biggest challenges facing the AAT and AAI fields: first, the feel-good assumption that dogs, in any context and with any patient, make everything better; and second, that you cannot take human-animal interaction seriously because it's "just about pets" and what is scientific about that? The answer to the latter is—a lot, thanks to the work and expertise of the authors of the book's chapters. Their chapters are rich with case examples, practical applications, and insights about what we know, as well as what we still need to know, to make progress in the field. This book will do much to advance the fields of AAT and AAI, to remind practitioners that the welfare of the animals involved must be protected, and to establish that companion animals, in the right context, can play a vital role in treating mental health illness and developmental disorders.

We are all "trapped in the well" to some degree, including mental health professionals who struggle to balance heavy patient loads with staying current about the best ways to help them. Some people are down deeper than others, and in some cases, as we learn in the pages that follow, there are indeed Lassies out there just waiting to assist in the rescue.

Patricia B. McConnell, Ph.D.

Certified Applied Animal Behaviorist
Author, *The Education of Will* and
The Other End of the Leash

1

Introduction

Nancy R. Gee, Ph.D.
Lisa D. Townsend, Ph.D., LCSW
Robert L. Findling, M.D., M.B.A.

HUMANS AND ANIMALS have led a shared existence for thousands of years, and through the ages we have come to find ways to coexist to the benefit of both humans and animals, although most benefits have accrued to humans. This is primarily because animals occupy many important roles in the lives of humans; animals are our companions, our workers, our assistants, and our resources. Our relationships with animals are ancient, and the bond we share can be deeply meaningful, yet our relationships with animals can also be fraught with complexities. For example, some animals are kept for companionship, others for food, and still others for specific jobs. Because animals do not speak a human language, humans struggle to understand their perspective and in many cases simply ignore it and treat animals as possessions or commodities, commonly assuming that they are not sentient and are bereft of emotion.

On the contrary, several animal species have demonstrated that they are sensitive to emotions and can discriminate emotional expressions and extract information from faces and vocalizations, and dogs specifically have shown that they can infer emotional states and use this information to make decisions (Albuquerque et al. 2022). Furthermore, the relationship people establish with their dogs may affect the degree to which their dogs are sensitive to the emotional states of their owners.

For example, one study showed that emotional states could be transferred from humans to dogs (emotional contagion), particularly female dogs, but the efficacy of the transfer was dependent on the duration of time shared between the human and the dog (Katayama et al. 2019). These results suggest that dogs can learn many social experiences from living with humans that may be formed by a long-term affiliative relationship or from acquired associations learned over time. Longer ownership may result in a tighter bond, fostering an oxytocin-mediated loop in which both the human and the dog benefit from oxytocin's facilitation of recognition of emotional states in others.

Dogs and humans have a long coevolutionary history, and their ability to communicate via visual and acoustic systems has been ascertained repeatedly (MacLean et al. 2017b). This interspecies communicative potential was extended to olfactory signals associated with fear and happiness in humans, which the dogs discriminated with near-perfect accuracy (D'Aniello et al. 2018). All of this indicates not only that dogs are keen observers of human behaviors, including displays of emotions, but also that dogs use their superior sense of smell to supplement the information they glean with their eyes and ears, which may give them an observational advantage over humans, even though they have not mastered the use of human languages. In addition to these key skills, dogs in particular appear hardwired to attach to those beings around them as they mature (see Wynne 2019 for a complete discussion of this idea), making them particularly well suited for bonding with humans. As the scientific study of human-animal interaction (HAI) grows, questions have emerged regarding the mechanisms underlying the observed effects. Several theoretical models have been formulated to answer these questions about the unique nature of some human-animal relationships.

Theoretical Perspectives on the Human-Animal Bond

The human-animal bond has been defined by the American Veterinary Medical Association (1998, p. 1675) as "a mutually beneficial and dynamic relationship between people and animals that is influenced by behaviors considered essential to the health and well-being of both. The bond includes, but is not limited to, the emotional, psychological, and physical interactions of people, animals, and the environment." The bond that we share with animals has been well documented and described in a wide variety of literatures, including ancient literature, modern fiction, and research reports in the professional literature (for a discussion of this literature and the human-animal bond, see Fine and Beck 2019). Several hypotheses, theories, and frameworks have been adapted or developed to conceptualize the effect of this bond on both people and animals. For example, the biophilia hypothesis describes humans as having an "innate tendency to focus on life and lifelike processes" (Wilson 1984, p. 1), making us uniquely drawn to animals and nature. Unfortunately, this hypothesis fails to provide predictive power in HAI research, but it is used routinely as a commonly accepted tenet for appreciating why humans may be motivated to interact with, and potentially develop attachments to, animals.

Attachment Theory

Attachment theory postulates that human infants develop a strong emotional connection with a primary attachment figure and display certain behaviors indicative of attachment (Bowlby 1969). Furthermore, children develop attachment relationships with others as they mature and establish specific attachment styles (Ainsworth 1993). Attachment theory has been used to describe human attachment to companion animals (Meehan et al. 2017). In Western households, the presence of companion animals is almost as common as that of siblings (Cassels et al. 2017). Many people consider their pets to be members of their families, and pets are reported to fulfill the four roles of attachment figures: enjoyable, comforting, missed when absent, and sought out in times of distress. Their nonjudgmental nature makes them a particularly valuable resource for communication among those who are low in self-disclosure or high in self-consciousness, adolescents (particularly boys who report disclosing less than girls do), and young and older adults (see Cassels et al. 2017 for a summary of this research). Considerable evidence supports a connection between attachment or caregiving and the oxytocin system (for a comprehensive review of this topic, see Julius et al. 2013), and the positive effects of HAI overlap with those of oxytocin. In fact, affiliative HAI has been found to stimulate the release of oxytocin, which has been shown to facilitate social behaviors and cognition (MacLean et al. 2017a). Furthermore, research has shown that dogs display similar attachment styles to their owners to those that human children display to their parents (Solomon et al. 2019). All of this indicates that attachment may be an important component in the human-animal bond and in the associated effects or benefits related to that bond.

Social Support Theory

The research on social support has been clustered into three perspectives that attempt to explain the effect of social support on human mental health (Lakey and Cohen 2000). First, social support reduces or buffers the effects of stress on health. Second, the perception of support, regardless of whether that perception matches the level of actual support from others, has been linked to positive health outcomes. Third, being in a relationship or relationships and experiencing companionship and intimacy are associated with positive health outcomes. As mentioned earlier, people often identify their companion animals as being an important part of their social networks (Meehan et al. 2017). Animals may provide nonjudgmental support by supplying a safe haven for physical comfort and communication without fear that the animal will disclose any confidences or betray trust, suggesting that having an animal participate in mental health therapy may have many follow-on effects that enhance that experience.

Biopsychosocial Model

For more than four decades, the biopsychosocial model (Figure 1–1) has been used to provide a framework for understanding how biological, psychological, and social influences may combine to determine human health and well-being (Engel 1980). Recently, the biopsychosocial model was used to contextualize a wide variety of research in HAI in which dogs were included as an adjunct to treatment or as a complementary therapy to improve some aspect of human health and well-being (Gee et al. 2021). A dynamic version of the model was used to organize findings and consider possible mechanisms of action. For example, interacting with a dog may affect human health and well-being through the mechanism of stress reduction, with biological effects coming in the form of decreased heart rate, blood pressure, and cortisol levels and increases in oxytocin levels. In the psychological realm, stress reduction has been seen in the form of almost immediate improvements in self-report measures of mood, stress, and anxiety. Finally, social effects of stress reduction may be found both immediately and over time in the form of improvements in social support networks, social development, and overall social health. The dynamic aspect of this model is seen in the timing of various effects and in the interrelation among the three realms, such that changes in the biological realm are likely to affect the psychological realm, and so on.

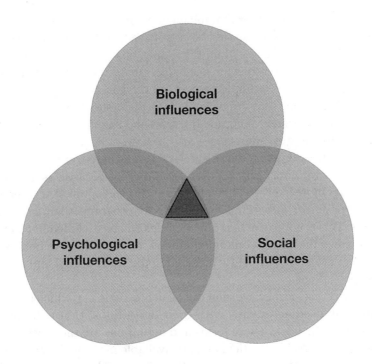

Figure 1–1. The three influences on human health in the biopsychosocial model.

What Is Ahead?

For some humans, animals are key attachment figures, beloved family members, and nonjudgmental partners sharing their journey through life. This volume is intended to represent the spectrum of relationships between people and their pets, highlighting both sides of the relationship and delineating the ways in which companion animals may be involved in the treatment of human mental illness. One of the key purposes of this book is to summarize what is known, as well as what is not known, about both the potential benefits and the potential risks of animal-based therapeutic intervention for persons with emotional and/or behavioral challenges.

Many people enjoy and derive benefit from interacting with animals. However, some individuals dislike interacting with animals, may be allergic to them, or may have a cultural or religious objection to them. Because people often openly state their preferences regarding companion animals, deciding whether to implement an animal-based intervention for an individual patient should be easy, based on their preferences.

All of this begs the question, What does this book offer the reader? In truth, one of the reasons for this book is to acknowledge that the decision about whether to implement an animal-based intervention is not always a simple one. It is important to fully understand the strength and quality of the evidence alongside the risks and benefits associated with various types of programs.

It is worth noting that the research presented herein and the ensuing discussions will most often center around dogs, because as a species they are far more likely to be involved in anthrozoology or HAI research, clinical practice, and animal-based activity programs than any other species. This is not to say that other species will be excluded but simply to recognize that of all nonhuman animal, or companion animal, species, dogs are more frequently included in the study of HAI and its various applications.

To start this journey, we refer the reader to Table 1–1, which includes commonly used acronyms, with their definitions, that will appear throughout the book. These terms and definitions are the most widely used and accepted in the field and are available in the white paper that is freely available in 19 languages on the website of the International Association of Human-Animal Interaction Organizations (2018). Also included in this important paper are clearly stated guidelines for human and animal well-being, including safety measures for both the human and the animal. Importantly, the white paper stipulates which animal species (domesticated species such as dogs, cats, and horses, with appropriate training and temperament) may be involved in animal-assisted activities (AAAs), animal-assisted therapy (AAT), and animal-assisted interventions (AAIs) and which animals are not appropriate (wild animal species such as dolphins, elephants, and capuchin monkeys).

Although the chapters that follow will present the science and best practices, including examples supporting the involvement of companion animals in the treatment of human mental illness, we would like to highlight an important theme running throughout this volume: respect for the animals involved and concern for their well-being. The first two chapters set the stage by focusing on dogs as partners in the treatment process. Chapter 2 (Fine) provides important information about ensuring canine welfare and well-being, identifying stressors, and providing guidance to clinicians to help them make good decisions about involving a dog in their work. Chapter 3 (Winkle and Jacaruso) further stresses the importance of animal welfare, while focusing on the different roles

Table 1–1. Commonly used terms and their accepted definitions according to the International Association of Human–Animal Interaction Organizations

Acronym	Term	Definition
AAA	Animal-assisted activity	"Informal interaction and visitation conducted by the human-animal team for motivational, educational and recreational purposes."
AAT	Animal-assisted therapy	"A goal oriented, planned and structured therapeutic intervention directed and/or delivered by health, education or human services professionals, including e.g. psychologists and social workers. Intervention progress is measured and included in professional documentation. AAT is delivered and/or directed by a formally trained (with active licensure, degree or equivalent) professional with expertise within the scope of the professionals' practice."
AAI	Animal-assisted intervention	"A goal oriented and structured intervention that intentionally includes or incorporates animals in health, education and human services (e.g., social work) for the purpose of therapeutic gains in humans. It involves people with knowledge of the people and animals involved. Animal assisted interventions incorporate human-animal teams in human services, such as Animal Assisted Therapy (AAT)."

Source. International Association of Human-Animal Interaction Organizations 2018, p. 5.

for animals in support of human mental health, with an emphasis on understanding applicable laws and regulations.

Chapters 4 through 13 follow the selective and indicated preventive intervention framework outlined by Mrazek and Haggerty (1994) in the Institute of Medicine report on reducing risk for mental disorders. Universal interventions are those recommended for the population as a whole and are considered to be beneficial for maintaining health and preventing disorder. Selective interventions address specific risk factors for illness and are provided for groups of people with greater biological, psychological, or environmental risk for disorder relative to others. Indicated interventions ameliorate risk factors associated with a high probability of disorder onset.

Chapters are organized using a life-course perspective within the selective/indicated intervention framework: Chapter 4 (Stewart and Hightower) reviews animal-assisted crisis interventions that are selectively provided for people who have experienced a significant trauma, such as a natural disaster, and are intended to prevent the onset of PTSD. Chapter 5 (Townsend and Mueller) highlights animal-assisted programs for youth at risk for mental disorders secondary to childhood maltreatment or who have a high likelihood of contact with the juvenile justice system. Disorder-specific, environment-specific, and life-stage-specific chapters (Chapters 6–13) begin with mental illnesses that typically present during childhood or adolescence and move through mental illnesses associated with older adulthood, including terminal illnesses. Beginning with Chapter 6 (Schuck and Childress), we move into disorder-specific AAAs, AAIs, and AATs designed to improve executive functioning, attention, and impulse control for youth with ADHD. Chapter 7 (O'Haire, Rodriguez, Neiforth, and Mao) introduces the reader to AAIs and AATs for people who have autism spectrum disorder, discussing ways to improve interpersonal communication and impulse control for those young people. Chapters 8 (Townsend, Gee, and Kornstein) and 9 (Friedmann, Gee, and Levenson) feature animal-assisted strategies for improving symptoms of major depressive disorder and anxiety disorders, highlighting how animal-assisted interactions can target intransigent symptoms such as anhedonia. Chapter 10 (Krause-Parello, Torres, Pratt, Moreno, and Hibler) highlights the role of animals in relieving symptoms of PTSD and illustrates how such interventions have been used with military veterans. Chapter 11 (Townsend and Buckley) introduces animal-assisted programs for people with schizophrenia and articulates the role of HAI in improving treatment-refractory negative symptoms such as low motivation and problems with social skills. Chapter 12 (Townsend) shows how animals can assist individuals and families in hospice care, highlighting how animals can ease pain and anxiety for patients reaching the end of life. HAIs in the context of aging, cognitive decline, and dementia are reviewed in Chapter 13 (Gee, Bibbo, and Dunn), focusing on how animals can soothe agitation for people with dementia and may slow declines in physical and mental health for older adults.

Following these content-focused chapters, we turn to three chapters that focus specifically on the application of HAI on university campuses (Chapter 14; Pendry, Milatz, Carr, and Vandagriff), in hospital settings (Chapter 15; Gee, Townsend, and Thakre), and in psychotherapy (Chapter 16; Chandler). The book concludes with a summary of what we know about the human-animal bond and its role in recovery from psychiatric illness and what we still need to learn. Threaded throughout the book is a focus on the intertwinement of human and animal well-being.

The Decision to Recommend a Pet to a Patient

Physicians and mental health providers are often asked by their patients and family members of patients about whether they recommend a pet to provide support for a given mental or physical health condition in one of these patients. A simple Google search (conducted March 19, 2022) on the words "dogs for ASD" produced 17.4 million hits, evidencing the sheer popularity of the idea that having a dog may be beneficial to children with autism spectrum disorder. This topic is discussed in more detail in Chapter 7, but the short answer is twofold: 1) the idea is popular among the animal-loving community, and 2) the existing evidence on the topic of the health benefits of pet ownership is not strong, so pet ownership recommendations do not yet have a clear basis. For example, some evidence indicates that owning a pet, particularly a dog, may be causally related to a reduced risk of cardiovascular disease (Levine et al. 2013). However, almost all of the research to date on pet ownership is correlational in nature, and it is not possible to infer causation. Generally speaking, pet owners prefer to select their own pets rather than having one randomly assigned to them for the purposes of a study. This results in an inherent selection bias, leaving us in the awkward position of not knowing whether owning a pet makes people healthier or if healthier people opt to own pets. The trends in pet ownership show a clear decline with advancing age, which mirrors a decline in physical and cognitive functioning (Friedmann et al. 2020), indicating that pet ownership may be linked with health status, but it is important to understand that this does not mean that pet ownership confers health status.

There has been much press on the idea that pets make us healthier. A recent Google search (also conducted March 19, 2022) using the words "do dogs make us healthier" resulted in 393 million hits. These stories cover a variety of topics, including the health benefits of pets, the ways that pets make humans happier, science-backed benefits of owning a pet, and health- and mood-boosting effects of pets. These stories are enjoyable to read and are clearly very popular with the general public, but an association between any health outcome and pet ownership status does not mean that owning a pet was the causal factor. As with all correlational outcomes, there are three possibilities: 1) pets make people healthier, 2) healthy people opt to own pets, or 3) other variables are driving both health and pet ownership status. The popularity of the idea that pets make us healthier does not make it true, and we encourage the reader to think very carefully before recommending pets to clients and, importantly, to consider the well-being of the animal alongside the demands that may be placed on the animal, realistic or otherwise, before making any such recommendation.

Risk Assessment

The decision to begin an animal-based therapeutic intervention does require careful consideration. Risk assessment is paramount when contemplating the incorporation of an animal into the treatment plan for a person with mental illness, or even into a general approach to improving one's mental health and well-being. There are a number of considerations from both the animal side and the human side of this dynamic. With regard to the animal: Will a therapy animal be able to be kept safe during the time with the patient? Will a companion animal be adequately tended to under the patient's care? From the human side of the process: Is the patient afraid of or allergic to the animal? How will the presence of an animal affect psychiatric treatment? Have measures been taken to reduce the risk of zoonotic disease transmission?

For our purposes, *risk assessment* refers to the process by which one identifies potential hazards or factors that may result in harm to either the human or the animal involved in the HAI. An important part of risk assessment involves developing specific approaches to mitigating all hazards identified. Although the Lincoln Education Assistance with Dogs (LEAD) Risk Assessment Tool was originally designed to be used in educational settings, it was also developed to be flexibly applied to a variety of AAI and AAA settings (Brelsford et al. 2020). The tool comprises several parts, including assessment details, hazard identification and control measures, an action plan, and a dog care plan. In Table 1–2, we provide a rough outline of how this tool can be modified for use in mental health settings.

Finally, it is important to assess the risks associated with recommending that someone acquire a pet, an emotional support animal, or a psychiatric service dog. For a detailed discussion of these issues, please see Chapter 3 ("Roles of Animals With Individuals Who Have Mental Illness") in this volume.

Diversity, Equity, and Inclusion Considerations

Animals play a vital role in the lives of humans. Science has only begun to explore the complexities of human-animal relationships and how the well-being of humans is intertwined with that of animals. It is important also to consider the human-animal bond within cultural and religious contexts, because great variability is seen in attitudes toward animals in relation to these factors (Jegatheesan 2019). Some commonly held ideas such as the sacred cow among Asian Indians or the idea that Muslims may view dogs as unclean may impede understanding of and appreciation for cultural and religious differences and potentially diminish thoughtful consideration of individual perspectives. Relationships with companion animals vary or are perhaps more complicated depending on several factors related to diversity, yet there is a glaring dearth of research on this topic (Risley-Curtiss et al. 2006).

Carey et al. (2022) used a nonrandomized controlled trial design to evaluate the effects of a therapy dog visit on pain, depression, and anxiety among patients in an emergency department waiting room. Although no differences were noted in outcomes across age, gender, or ethnicity, it is important to note that the majority of patients (82.3%) identified as white. Risley-Curtiss et al. (2006) examined the relationship between pet ownership and race/ethnicity in a random sample of people living in the United States. The overall ethnic breakout of pet ownership indicated that participants who self-identified as American Indian were most likely to have pets (74%), followed by people who identified as white (65%), Hispanic/Spanish (57%), African American (41%), Pacific Islander (40%), and Asian (38%). In terms of types of pets owned, dogs were the most commonly owned pet (79% of sample). People who identified as Hispanic/Spanish were significantly less likely to have cats or birds, and people who identified as American Indian were more likely to have fish; otherwise, there were no significant differences across ethnic groups for types of animals owned. These studies illustrate two important points:

Table 1–2. **Rough outline for modifying the Lincoln Education Assistance with Dogs (LEAD) Risk Assessment Tool (Brelsford et al. 2020) for use in mental health settings**

Assessment details	Facility/location/address
	People involved (e.g., participants, animal handlers)
	People who oversee (e.g., administrators)
	People who need to be informed (e.g., parent/ guardian, other health care provider, medical power of attorney)
	Contact information for all
	Emergency contact numbers
	Incident contact numbers
Hazard identification	Examples include but are not limited to the following:
	Zoonotic disease
	Allergies
	Parasites
	Phobias
	Potential for aggression or abuse
	Environmental hazards
Control measures	Examples include but are not limited to the following:
	Adherence to established facility safety policies and protocols should be ensured.
	Hand sanitizer should be used before and after petting the dog.
	Dogs should undergo routine veterinary examination and be current on all vaccines.
	Dogs should be receiving flea and tick prevention measures.
	Participants should be screened for allergies, phobias, and potential for aggression.
	The environment should be examined closely for anything that may be harmful to a dog (e.g., a swinging door that may catch a paw or tail), and handlers should be directed around those potential hazards (e.g., have them use a different door) or alerted to them and given instructions on how to safely navigate the environment.

Table 1–2. **Rough outline for modifying the Lincoln Education Assistance with Dogs (LEAD) Risk Assessment Tool (Brelsford et al. 2020) for use in mental health settings *(continued)***

Action plan	Identify a responsible party to undertake the following:
	Ongoing assessment of people/animals/ environment to identify any additional hazards not previously identified
	Steps to mitigate/control newly identified hazards
	Ongoing evaluation of efficacy of all control measures
Dog care plan	The dog care plan in the LEAD Risk Assessment Tool can readily be applied to animal-assisted intervention situations without alteration. For animal-assisted therapy situations, additional considerations must be included, such as the following:
	An individualized working schedule must be determined for each dog (dogs may work more than 2 hours per day, but additional behavioral evaluation and independent monitoring are required).
	Scheduled exercise and sleep breaks need to be developed according to the individual animal's needs.
	Rules of interaction need to be agreed on in advance with each client to protect the dog during the sessions.

1) although study samples may be representative of the general U.S. population, findings may not generalize to specific cultural or ethnic subgroups; and 2) many people from racial/ethnic minority backgrounds have companion animals. HAI research must begin to incorporate a specific focus on underrepresented groups; their relationships with companion animals; and how AAAs, AAIs, and AAT can best meet their needs.

More than 65% of adults who identify as LGBTQ+ own pets, and older LGBTQ+ adults who own pets report higher perceived social support (Matijczak et al. 2020). Although pet ownership may be beneficial to marginalized groups, some evidence suggests that pet ownership may be related to aspects of privilege. For example, in a nationally representative cohort of older adults (50 years or older) living in the United States, pet ownership was associated with higher socioeconomic status (Shieu et al. 2022). Crossman and Kazdin (2018) discuss the theory of "destigmatization by association." This theory posits that because people generally have positive attitudes toward companion animals, those attitudes may "rub off" on the person they are seen with. The implication is that owning a pet may be beneficial for ethnic minorities or people of marginalized groups, who are perceived, when accompanied by a companion animal, in a better light than they may have been otherwise.

Conclusion

This book introduces the reader to the latest research on the role that animals can play in recovery from psychiatric illness as well as emerging work on the biological and psychological mechanisms underlying the human-animal bond. In an era when evidence-based treatments and empiricism are key principles in delivering care, an appreciation and understanding about what can be expected from an animal-based intervention can allow providers, patients, and their families to make informed decisions about whether an animal-based intervention is possibly appropriate for a given individual. This book summarizes the extant knowledge while highlighting what is not yet known about animal-based interventions in particular patient groups. In addition, this book focuses on key principles and considerations that are used when deciding whether an animal-based intervention might be appropriate for a given patient.

In this book, we address practical considerations for implementing animal-assisted programs in mental health and hospital contexts and provide useful tools for program planning. Our goal is to provide a scientifically grounded review of the research on HAIs and recovery from mental illness and inspire the reader to consider the role that animals play in ameliorating psychiatric symptoms, engaging patients in treatment, and enhancing well-being. Finally, we hope to leave the reader with a strong sense of our individual and global responsibility for considering animal well-being and the potential importance of the human-animal bond in the treatment of mental illness and promotion of mental health.

References

Ainsworth MS: Attachment as related to mother-infant interaction. Advances in Infancy Research 8:1–50, 1993

Albuquerque N, Mills DS, Guo K, et al: Dogs can infer implicit information from human emotional expressions. Anim Cogn 25(2):231–240, 2022 34390430

American Veterinary Medical Association: Statement from the Committee on the Human-Animal Bond. J Am Vet Med Assoc 212(11):1675, 1998

Bowlby J: Attachment and Loss, Vol 1: Attachment. New York, Basic Books, 1969

Brelsford VL, Dimolareva M, Gee NR, Meints K: Best practice standards in animal-assisted interventions: how the LEAD Risk Assessment Tool can help. Animals (Basel) 10(6):974, 2020 32503309

Carey B, Dell CA, Stempien J, et al: Outcomes of a controlled trial with visiting therapy dog teams on pain in adults in an emergency department. PLoS One 17(3):e0262599, 2022 35263346

Cassels MT, White N, Gee N, Hughes C: One of the family? Measuring young adolescents' relationships with pets and siblings. J Appl Dev Psychol 49:12–20, 2017

Crossman MK, Kazdin AE: Perceptions of animal-assisted interventions: the influence of attitudes toward companion animals. J Clin Psychol 74(4):566–578, 2018 29023782

D'Aniello B, Semin GR, Alterisio A, et al: Interspecies transmission of emotional information via chemosignals: from humans to dogs (Canis lupus familiaris). Anim Cogn 21(1):67–78, 2018 28988316

Engel GL: The clinical application of the biopsychosocial model. Am J Psychiatry 137(5):535–544, 1980 7369396

Fine AH, Beck AM: Understanding our kinship with animals: input for health care professionals interested in the human-animal bond, in Animal-Assisted Therapy: Foundations and Guidelines for Animal-Assisted Interventions, 5th Edition. Edited by Fine AH. London, Elsevier Academic Press, 2019, pp 3–12

Friedmann E, Gee NR, Simonsick EM, et al: Pet ownership patterns and successful aging outcomes in community dwelling older adults. Front Vet Sci 7:293, 2020 32671105

Gee NR, Rodriguez KE, Fine AH, Trammell JP: Dogs supporting human health and well-being: a biopsychosocial approach. Front Vet Sci 8:630465, 2021 33860004

International Association of Human-Animal Interaction Organizations: The IAHAIO Definitions for Animal Assisted Intervention and Guidelines for Wellness of Animals Involved in AAI. 2014, updated April 2018. Available at: https://iahaio.org/wp/wp-content/uploads/2021/01/iahaio-white-paper-2018-english.pdf. Accessed August 2, 2022.

Jegatheesan B: Influence of cultural and religious factors on attitudes towards animals, in Animal-Assisted Therapy: Foundations and Guidelines for Animal-Assisted Interventions, 5th Edition. Edited by Fine AH. London, Elsevier Academic Press, 2019, pp 43–49

Julius H, Beetz A, Kotrschal K, et al: Attachment to Pets: An Integrative View of Human-Animal Relationships With Implications for Therapeutic Practice. Cambridge, MA, Hogrefe Publishing, 2013

Katayama M, Kubo T, Yamakawa T, et al: Emotional contagion from humans to dogs is facilitated by duration of ownership. Front Psychol 10:1678, 2019 31379690

Lakey B, Cohen S: Social support theory and measurement, in Social Support Measurement and Intervention: A Guide for Health and Social Scientists. Edited by Cohen S, Underwood LG, Gottlieb BH. New York, Oxford University Press, 2000, pp 29–52

Levine GN, Allen K, Braun LT, et al; American Heart Association Council on Clinical Cardiology; Council on Cardiovascular and Stroke Nursing: Pet ownership and cardiovascular risk: a scientific statement from the American Heart Association. Circulation 127(23):2353–2363, 2013 23661721

MacLean EL, Gesquiere LR, Gee NR, et al: Effects of affiliative human–animal interaction on dog salivary and plasma oxytocin and vasopressin. Front Psychol 8:1606, 2017a 28979224

MacLean EL, Herrmann E, Suchindran S, Hare B: Individual differences in cooperative communicative skills are more similar between dogs and humans than chimpanzees. Anim Behav 126:41–51, 2017b

Matijczak A, McDonald SE, Tomlinson CA, et al: The moderating effect of comfort from companion animals and social support on the relationship between microaggressions and mental health in LGBTQ+ emerging adults. Behav Sci (Basel) 11(1):1, 2020 33374678

Meehan M, Massavelli B, Pachana N: Using attachment theory and social support theory to examine and measure pets as sources of social support and attachment figures. Anthrozoos 30(2):273–289, 2017

Mrazek PJ, Haggerty RJ; Committee on Prevention of Mental Disorders, Institute of Medicine: Reducing Risks for Mental Disorders: Frontiers for Preventive Intervention Research. Washington, DC, National Academy Press, 1994, p 21

Risley-Curtiss C, Holley LC, Wolf S: The animal-human bond and ethnic diversity. Soc Work 51(3):257–268, 2006 17076123

Shieu M, Applebaum J, Dunietz G, Braley T: Companion animals and cognitive health: a population-based study. Neurology 98(18 Suppl):671, 2022

Solomon J, Beetz A, Schöberl I, et al: Attachment security in companion dogs: adaptation of Ainsworth's strange situation and classification procedures to dogs and their human caregivers. Attach Hum Dev 21(4):389–417, 2019 30246604

Wilson EO: Biophilia: The Human Bond With Other Species. Cambridge, MA, Harvard University Press, 1984

Wynne CD: Dog Is Love: Why and How Your Dog Loves You. Boston, MA, Houghton Mifflin, 2019

2

A Working Partnership Between Clinicians and Therapy Dogs in the Treatment of Mental Disorders

Aubrey H. Fine, Ed.D.

OVER THE PAST several decades, the use of animal-assisted interventions (AAIs) has gone from a marginalized field to an accepted complementary therapy (Fine et al. 2019a, 2019b). Most of the early scientific investigations in the field of human-animal interaction (HAI) focused on the ways that animals have contributed to the well-being of humans. The research is also filled with results highlighting the physiological and psychological benefits of the bond in humans (Fine et al. 2019a). Nevertheless, until recently there has been a lack of rigorous, repeatable re-

---

The author would like to thank Stefanie Malzyner for her research assistance in the preparation of this chapter. An additional thank-you is given to John Ugalidi for his efforts in reviewing this chapter and providing editorial suggestions.

search showing the efficacy of AAIs (Fine et al. 2019a, 2019b). That is now changing with an emergent body of new higher-quality research that more reliably assesses the effect of AAIs.

Although a wide variety of animals are engaged in AAIs, I focus primarily on dogs, the species most likely to be found in clinical settings (Brodie et al. 2002). For the reasons cited below, the relationship between humans and dogs makes them uniquely well suited to serve as therapeutic adjuncts.

Huls (2021) highlighted the value of daily HAI. He cited two interviews with leading academics in the field (Drs. Eric Strauss and Clive Winn), who agreed that dogs and humans see the world in remarkably similar ways. Both researchers suggested that there is no other animal with which people have had a stronger relationship than with dogs. Historically, anthropologists and other social scientists can trace human interactions with dogs back 15,000–30,000 years (Benz-Schwarzburg et al. 2020). The details explaining the domestication of dogs remain unclear, although Miklósi and Topál (2013) suggested that specific wolves were selected for domestication by humans primarily because of their cooperation and communication skills. Many contemporary species of dogs have a genetic predisposition toward both of these traits. The evolutionary changes that we now witness in the modern-day dog developed in the canid's brain over a long time. Kaminski and Marshall-Pescini (2014) explained that these changes were due to the expansion of the dog's prorean gyrus at the anterior end of the neocortex and a general increase in the amount of infoldings of the frontal lobe, in addition to an expansion of the prefrontal cortex.

Anthropologists and zoologists may differ on how the human-canine relationship was forged over time, but most agree that it was mutually established. The trust built between humans and dogs was a gradual process that seemed to begin with each supporting the other. The dogs appeared to initially associate humans with being their consistent source of food. From their vantage point, spending time in the proximity of humans meant getting access to their food (usually leftovers or refuse) and water. While being around humans, the dogs were able to learn and understand humans' behaviors. In return, the dogs probably alerted the humans to the presence of other, potentially more dangerous predators, by defending their scraps. In essence, what transpired was the development of an early reciprocal relationship between people and dogs. Contemporary researchers and evolutionary anthropologists generally agree that dogs have become uniquely calibrated to live alongside humans (Huls 2021).

The Need for Clinicians to Understand Canine Welfare Issues

Most human health care providers have limited, or no, training in animal ethology and behavior. This lack of knowledge may directly affect awareness of, and sensitivity to, dog behavior and cognition and thus the ability to preserve and protect the welfare of the animals involved. It is incumbent on all practitioners to appreciate that the focus in HAI cannot be only on the human side of the equation. Clinicians also must appreciate the effect of AAIs on the animals that work with them.

In short, dogs are not humans in fur. They may see the world similarly, but they may respond differently during AAIs because of their canine behavioral makeup. Ensuring the welfare of the animals does not simply benefit the animals; it is essential to the overall efficacy of the entire AAI process (Peralta and Fine 2021a). By promoting good animal welfare practices, professionals will ensure that the partnerships will be more sustainable over time.

Animal Welfare: The Five Freedoms and Five Domains

Although organizations dedicated to preventing animal cruelty emerged in the nineteenth century, ensuring the well-being of domestic animals was not considered a priority on a global basis until the 1960s. A document entitled "Five Freedoms" (Peralta and Fine 2021a) emerged in 1965 from the United Kingdom's Farm Animal Welfare Council, a government animal care committee, and is considered to be the first major attempt to address and protect the well-being of livestock. The Five Freedoms identify freedoms and opportunities that farm animals should be given to enhance their well-being. They include freedom from hunger and thirst; freedom from discomfort; freedom from pain, injury, or disease; freedom to express normal behavior; and freedom from fear and distress (Peralta and Fine 2021b). Although the Five Freedoms have a broad use, they focus primarily on minimizing negative life outcomes rather than promoting optimal living.

In the mid-1990s, an alternative perspective known as the Five Domains emerged (Mellor and Beausoleil 2015). Although it parallels the Five Freedoms, the Five Domains model presents a two-tiered model clearly addressing both physical and mental states. It introduces a shift in orientation toward the promotion of positive states rather than simply the satisfaction of basic needs. The model emphasizes various life opportunities that lead to a positive affective state and an animal's perceived well-being (Mellor and Beausoleil 2015; Mellor et al. 2020). One of the most significant attributes of this model is the attempt to evaluate how HAIs affect animal welfare, and it emphasizes the responsibilities of humans to support their animals rather than negate their animals' behaviors. Figure 2–1 illustrates the elements within the Five Domains and areas that should be avoided.

Some elements within the Five Domains are easily affected during any HAI, and more specifically in AAIs. For example, the domain of Nutrition can be affected when any individual, including a client, unintentionally overfeeds a therapy animal thinking that food shows love and would enhance their relationship. In terms of Environment, to fulfill humans' needs, dogs may be taken to locations where they do not feel comfortable, perhaps because the location is crowded or requires an elevator ride. By considering the Five Domains model, clinicians can become more conscious of an animal's well-being and attempt to promote more opportunities to improve the animal's quality of life.

Canine Attributes Contributing to Effective Animal-Assisted Interventions

Various theories have been proposed to explain why dogs seem to seek out humans and are willing to help them in a time of need. Some believe that this outcome has developed over the period of domestication and now has neurobiological components. Others suggest that emotional contagion or synchronized emotions are relevant to this discussion. It is important to appreciate that dogs relate to the world around them differently than humans do. The term *umwelt* can be used to describe how animals perceive that world and how they use their senses differently than humans do (Uexkull 1957). For example, although dogs' vision may be of lower resolution than human vision, their abilities to smell and to hear are profoundly better than our own (Horowitz 2016).

Domestication

Miklósi and Topál (2013) have argued that the unique qualities of cooperation and communication that caused dogs to connect with humans initially may have resulted in a special sensitivity to human gestures,

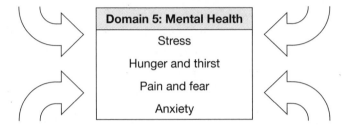

Domain 1: Nutrition	Domain 2: Environment
• Limited access to food and water • Excessive amounts of food	• Overstimulated living environment that is cold and noisy • The environment is unkept and disorderly. Food may be left for a long time and may be unsanitary.

Domain 5: Mental Health

Stress

Hunger and thirst

Pain and fear

Anxiety

Domain 3: Health	Domain 4: Behavior
• Poor preventive health care • Physically demanding interactions	• Being in harness with limited mobility • Being required to perform arduous inappropriate tasks

Figure 2–1. Five Domains model.

Source.   Adapted from the original Five Domains model of Mellor et al. 2009.

speech, and behavior. Research studies have highlighted the extent to which dogs can reliably observe and follow a large set of basic human cues, helping them to better understand what humans expect of them (Udell et al. 2008). Some researchers (Müller et al. 2015; Ruffman and Morris-Trainor 2011) suggest that this ability is enhanced because the dogs' visual skills help them assess the various emotional states displayed by humans.

Emotional Contagion

Emotional contagion or emotional state matching refers to an individual's ability to mirror another's behavior and therefore prompt an empathetic response. Research has shown that animals ranging from primates to rodents can demonstrate emotional contagion. Dogs have been found to distinguish different emotional expressions in human faces (Huber et al. 2017; Müller et al. 2015) and produce a facial mimicry response in less than 1 second (Palagi et al. 2015). Dogs not only can recognize dog and human emotions but also can categorize others' emotions, which facilitates information processing and their ability to comprehend what others are portraying and how they are feeling (Albuquerque et al. 2016).

That said, because of this expertise, dogs seem capable of conveying comfort-offering behaviors to their human companions. In a study by Custance and Mayer (2012), dogs had an empathetic response to hearing their humans pretending to cry. On analysis, the authors concluded that dogs did not show an understanding that the cry was a need for help, but rather exhibited an instance of emotional contagion. A study by Yong and Ruffman (2014) in which domestic dogs were confronted with infants crying, infants babbling, or white noise produced conflicting results. Of the three conditions, dogs expressed an empathetic response and were more alert only when hearing infant cries. The dogs also had increased cortisol levels similar to those produced by humans in comparable circumstances. These findings suggest that dogs can show primitive emotional contagion responses when confronted with human distress.

Canine Cognition

Researchers have made great progress toward understanding canine cognition in recent years, reporting that dogs are capable of understanding human words. In recent imaging studies, dogs' brains were found to respond to actual words, not just the tone in which they were recited (Andics et al. 2016). Miklósi and Kubinyi (2016) reported that some dogs are capable of recognizing more than 1,000 human words.

Therapy Dogs: Stress in Their Workplace

Results and opinions about whether therapy dogs experience stress during AAIs differ. Careful initial selection of therapy dogs and proper training and handling may be key factors, although it is always possible that unique circumstances can trigger unanticipated reactions in therapy dogs.

Several studies have concluded that the work of a therapy dog can cause stress and discomfort in the animal. Haubenhofer and Kirchengast (2006, 2007) reported that more than 50% of handlers volunteering with their therapy dogs believed that AAI sessions may cause some stress for their dog. Their findings (from collected saliva samples and questionnaires) highlighted that therapy dogs had an increased level of salivary cortisol on the days that they were working in comparison to their nonworking days. Their reported findings also suggested that the cortisol level increased when the dogs worked in more sessions without ample time to recover. By contrast, Corsetti et al. (2019) determined that dogs observed in AAIs did not show significant increases in stress behaviors while interacting with humans. Their findings are consistent with research by McCullough et al. (2018) on the physiological and behavioral effects of AAIs on therapy dogs in pediatric oncology settings. Those authors did not find any consequential increase in stress, especially when the expectations were realistic and the dogs were well supervised. Similar results were found by Glenk et al. (2013), indicating that both therapy dogs in training and fully trained dogs did not show significantly increased levels of stress as assessed by their salivary cortisol levels during group therapy sessions when compared with nonworking levels.

It is possible to interpret this disparity in results with the argument that when therapy animals are selected appropriately, well trained, and well supervised, there may be less likelihood of stressing the animal. Similar findings were noted by van Houtert et al. (2021) in their research in the training of service dogs. Nevertheless, even though therapy dogs are typically selected and registered because of their behavioral consistency, temperament, and affiliative natures, some of the dogs still may show behaviors indicative of stress (known as "calming signs") in certain circumstances (Fine et al. 2013). Calming signs include panting, pacing, startle responses, pupillary dilation, trembling, whining, excessive licking, and yawning. It is incumbent on clinicians to appreciate that even a trained therapy dog may feel uncomfortable at times for any number of reasons and that the clinician will need to respond appropriately to reduce the dog's discomfort.

When these behaviors are observed, clinicians must consider which antecedent factors may have contributed to the dog's stress (Fine et al. 2013; Ng and Fine 2021). Such factors could include the effect of the client's behavior, the effect of unusual environmental factors or stimuli, and the effect of therapist/handler behaviors on the interactions. A poor fit between job expectations and the selected dog may create an uncomfortable situation for all involved, especially the animal (Heimlich 2001).

Ng and Fine (2019, 2021) provide illustrations of these four factors that can help clinicians better understand the behavior of therapy dogs under specific circumstances. For example, therapy dogs may be asked to work with clients who have erratic behaviors. Unpredictable behaviors (such as screaming), as well as improper handling by the handler/clinician, may result in the therapy dog experiencing stress (Hall et al.

2019). Additionally, the simple novelty of working in changing environments (which may include the presence of unfamiliar sounds and odors) could be a source of significant stress for working dogs (Rooney et al. 2016). Ng et al. (2014) reported that therapy dogs exposed to a new working environment seemed to show signs of stress. The dogs' cortisol levels were significantly higher after 30 minutes when compared with the baseline data.

Therapy dogs' attachment to their handlers also may play a role. The behavior of a dog may differ when the animal is in the presence of, and working with, an individual to whom they are securely attached (Fatjó et al. 2021). Wanser and Udell (2019) observed that dogs who were not securely attached showed a difference in their eye contact with their handlers (in comparison to those dogs who were attached to their handlers). Mills et al. (2013) found that dogs were more willing to interact in a novel environment when their secure individual was in that environment with them. Fine (2019) asserted that when this relationship is solidified, the interactions between the dog and the clinician can become more fluid and seamless.

Glenk et al. (2013) suggested that a potential way to decrease the dog's stress is for the handler/clinician to offer more flexibility in what is expected of the dog during visitations and to avoid additional engagements if the dog does not appear to enjoy the process. In other words, dogs, like people, respond better when allowed agency over their behaviors.

Guidelines for Initial Selection of Therapy Dogs

AAI literature has begun to produce agreed-on guidelines for selecting dogs well suited to work as therapy dogs.

Age

King et al. (2011), in their research, found that therapy dogs younger than 2 years showed more signs of stress than therapy dogs who were older and had more experience. Their research illustrated significant elevations in canine salivary cortisol levels in 21 younger dogs from baseline to after 1 hour of an AAI in a hospital environment (King et al. 2011).

Life Balance

King et al.'s findings, as well as the work of others (Ng and Fine 2019; Peralta and Fine 2021b), highlighted that dogs need to have a healthy balance of other activities in their lives beyond being engaged in AAIs. This balance should include proper additional outlets for outside play and relaxation, in addition to allowing the dogs the time to mature before they are engaged in work settings.

Selecting the Right Dog for the Correct Job

Although it is now accepted (see Peralta and Fine 2021a; Svartberg 2006) that we must ensure that dogs selected to work in any given environment show consistent and reliable behaviors, positive temperament, and an affiliative nature, the selection is actually more layered. We must appreciate that not all animals are suited for interactions in specific settings that have distinct purposes (MacNamara et al. 2019). For example, some dogs may work better with children than with adults. There is a need to develop clear guidelines for what should be expected in any workplace before a therapy dog is selected for the job. VanFleet et al. (2019) emphasized the concept of goodness of fit as one way to assess the expectations for the animal's engagement.

The Need for Proper Supervision

In regard to preventing stress in therapy dogs, attention must be given to ensuring proper supervision and appropriate engagement. For example, Melco et al. (2020) conducted a study evaluating the physiological effect of therapy work on registered dogs participating in a program with children with ADHD. The dogs involved in the study had minimal behavioral reactions and no significant changes in their cortisol levels or heart rate while in the program. The authors concluded that when stringent guidelines are put into place and the dog's welfare is strongly preserved, the overall outcome is positive.

Therapeutic Alliance

The presence of therapy dogs in various settings has a tremendous effect on enhancing the clinician-client relationship, or the therapeutic alliance (Dell et al. 2021; Fine 2019; López-Cepero 2020). Many factors can contribute to this alliance, including aspects of the client such as gender, race, and age. Nevertheless, it is evident that therapy animals make significant contributions to the therapeutic alliance (Meier et al. 2006). Studies have consistently found that the quality of the therapeutic alliance influences treatment outcomes (Orlinsky et al. 2003). The animal's presence can soften the discussion of an uncomfortable subject and support the client in disclosing their feelings. In fact, in a meta-analytic review of 11 studies on the relationship between psychotherapy dropout and therapeutic alliance in adult individual psychotherapy, the researchers found that clients with a weaker therapeutic alliance were more likely to drop out and discontinue psychotherapy (Sharf et al. 2010).

Furthermore, the animal's presence can reduce the client's anxiety and have an effect on their resistance to the therapeutic intervention (Chandler 2017; Fine 2019). Fine (2019) has often stressed that the animal's presence allows the clinician to go under the radar of the client's defense mechanisms. The clients seem to become more at ease, especially when the clinician and the therapy dog work in synchronized tandem. When this process works well, the client's bond with the animal has a positive effect on their commitment to fulfilling the therapeutic goals (Cieslak 2001).

The animal's presence in the environment has a strong effect on how the therapy is perceived (Fine 2019). The animal makes the environment appear safe and more comfortable. Flynn et al. (2020) reported the findings from 23 semistructured interviews with providers working at Green Chimneys, a nature-based therapeutic environment. Most of the respondents reported that the environment seemed to make the clients feel safer, supported, and not judged. They believed that the therapeutic milieu promoted a more comfortable workspace that supported the therapeutic process. They also believed that the working environment appeared much less threatening to the clients in comparison to those who received therapy in more traditional settings. Ultimately, it is apparent that a therapeutic environment that has animals present can be a viable alternative to traditional therapy, especially when the animals' involvement is planned and thought through.

Contraindications to Human-Animal Interaction and Animal-Assisted Interventions: Areas to Consider

Although HAI and AAIs can make valuable contributions to the well-being of human mental health, some negative outcomes and circumstances are possible. Two contraindications are the possibility of zoonosis (the transfer of disease from animals to humans) and the inability to ensure the safety of both animals and humans (such as in circumstances of animal abuse and animal hoarding).

Zoonosis

Animals that participate in AAI programs must be kept in excellent health for a variety of reasons (Fatjó et al. 2021). Keeping the animals healthy not only supports their own welfare but also reduces public health concerns. Clinicians engaged in AAIs should become much more aware of the zoonotic risks that could occur while working around therapy animals. One resource that may be helpful to review is the document published by the Society for Healthcare Epidemiology of America (Murthy et al. 2015). The document provides guidelines and recommendations for safely integrating AAIs in hospital settings. These recommendations focus on reducing the potential risks associated with having animals work in health care settings. Consequently, understanding the possibility of zoonosis is important for any professional working in this field or recommending such opportunities. For example, practitioners should become aware of common zoonotic diseases, including endoparasites (such as *Toxocara canis* in dogs) and other parasitic infections. Unfortunately, one possible challenge is that the working therapy dogs may act as fomites and carry infections between clients. This can be easily avoided if proper preventive measures are put into place (such as using hand sanitizer). Ultimately, all therapy animals should be monitored and treated for any emerging zoonotic diseases so that all humans can remain safe and healthy (Maurelli et al. 2019). Having a plan in place guarantees the health of the animals and consequently public health. Chur-Hansen et al. (2014) provided numerous suggestions to avoid zoonotic concerns. For example, they stressed that animals fed raw meat in the last 90 days should be excluded from AAI work.

In essence, practitioners must exercise due diligence by remaining conscious of zoonosis and its implications; they should strive to implement best practices with safety protocols in place to ensure good hygiene practices, including handwashing. When this effort is undertaken, the well-being of all involved will be better ensured.

Animal Abuse

Over the past few decades, some mental health providers have been keenly interested in providing support for people who have been accused of abusing animals. Abusing animals is now clearly seen as overlapping areas of child maltreatment, child abuse, domestic violence, and elder abuse (Arkow 2019; Finkelstein 2003). One disorder that may be overlooked as a potential signal of animal abuse is factitious disorder imposed on another. The disorder, also known as Munchausen syndrome by proxy, is quite a rare psychological disorder, with fewer than 1,000 cases reported annually. An individual with this disorder may falsely claim that a child in their care has, or may even inflict on the child, an illness or an injury because of the person's need to receive sympathy and attention. This disorder occurs not only between a parent and a child but also between owners and their pets. There are only a handful of cases highlighting this disorder in the victimization of pets (Oxley and Feldman 2016), but as is the case with parent/child abuse, the outcome of the falsification still relates to the need for personal gratification in the owner. Over the years, people may have either inflicted injuries on an animal or falsified them so that they could gain attention. For example, an individual may make false claims about the health of a pet to get continued sympathies from a veterinarian. They also may deprive the animal of sufficient food and sustenance so that they can have an excuse to get support and attention. This form of animal abuse must be monitored and understood by various clinicians. Mental health professionals as well as veterinarians need to be cognizant of this disorder, able to recognize it, and willing to intervene on behalf of the animals involved. Animals in these cases are like very young children, in that they need an advocate who will speak for them. It is incumbent on clinicians to take this role.

Animal Hoarding

According to the Hoarding of Animals Research Consortium (2002), animal hoarding "is characterized by an accumulation of an unusually large number of animals, failure to provide adequate care and living environment for the animals, and impairment in health, safety, and social or occupational functioning." Arluke and Patronek (2016) argue that animal hoarding is a more severe case of hoarding than other forms of object collecting. They believe that the significance can be more strongly manifested because of the emotional responses and the affection provided by the animals to the person.

Many animal hoarders live in very unhealthy environments that may include living in filth along with dead animals (Arkow 2019). Severe cases of hoarding endanger the health and safety of not only the hoarder and the animals but also the surrounding communities (Frost 2000; Frost et al. 2000). Although the subject of animal hoarding has not been extensively reviewed and studied, the outcome of not intervening early and providing support has detrimental effects on the well-being of the hoarder and the animals.

Hoarding of animals transcends gender, age, race, and socioeconomic status (Patronek 2001). Nevertheless, there do appear to be a disproportionate number of older women who hoard animals. These women also seem to be more socially isolated. However, the reason for such a significant difference between the genders remains unclear (Patronek and Nathanson 2009). Furthermore, older hoarders are at greater risk for zoonotic diseases, especially those with vulnerable immune systems (Reinisch 2008). For example, ammonia—which is present in animal urine—can, at high concentrations, lead to ocular and respiratory irritation.

Although many animal hoarders seem to have the right intentions or reasons for accumulating pets, the reality remains that many of these animals may end up being seriously neglected, as well as living in unsanitary conditions (Patronek 2001). The Hoarding of Animals Research Consortium (2002) identified four distinct types of animal hoarders (Patronek et al. 2006). Readers are encouraged to review the document for more details about the following subtypes: 1) hoarders with mental health issues, 2) overwhelmed caregivers, 3) rescuers, and 4) exploiters.

The most significant challenge in treating animal hoarding is that simply removing animals from a residence does not solve the problem. Treating hoarders is quite complicated, and many need psychological services and supports for recovery. With a 50% relapse rate, this deep-rooted psychiatric disorder is not sufficiently resolved by removing animals from homes (Reinisch 2008). There has been limited success with various forms of behavioral intervention in reducing the recidivism of animal hoarding, with 60%–100% of people continuing to have difficulties after being initially treated (Ockenden et al. 2014). Collaboration among various social service agencies serving both humans and animals is crucial in efforts to prevent animal hoarding (Reinisch 2008). It is imperative for clinicians to recognize and understand this medical condition so that we can potentially improve the lives of hoarders, animals, and their surrounding communities.

Conclusion

HAI and AAIs can be a viable option in supporting the psychosocial needs of individuals with various mental illnesses. It behooves interested providers to become aware of the mechanisms influenced by HAI and how the nature of canines can make the difference. These contributions can be significant, especially when attention is given to better understanding how these interactions may be meaningful. The interactions also must be carefully integrated into the overall treatment plan for the various individuals. Although HAI is a valuable option for many, clinicians also must be aware of contraindications for HAI, including the possibility of zoonosis, safety concerns with specific populations, and concerns about the welfare of the animals.

An unknown author is credited with the following quotation: "One reason a dog can be such a comfort when you're feeling blue is that s/he doesn't try to find out why. They never really ask questions, but they simply are ready to respond with needed comfort that may help." The essence of this comment may capture the true rationale for AAIs. These intentional acts of support with guided clinical direction may have a tremendous influence on the quality of life for many.

Key Clinical Points

- Human-animal interactions (HAIs) and animal-assisted interventions can be a viable option in supporting the psychosocial needs of individuals with various mental illnesses.

- Clinicians must be aware of contraindications for HAI, including the prospect of zoonosis, safety concerns with specific populations, and welfare concerns for the animals.

- Clinicians must understand how dogs respond differently to interactions than humans do because of their canine behaviors.

- Good welfare for the animals benefits not only the animals but also the overall efficacy of the entire process.

- The presence of therapy dogs in various settings has a tremendous effect on enhancing therapeutic alliance.

References

Albuquerque N, Guo K, Wilkinson A, et al: Dogs recognize dog and human emotions. Biol Lett 12(1):20150883, 2016 26763220

Andics A, Gábor A, Gácsi M, et al: Neural mechanisms for lexical processing in dogs. Science 353(6303):1030–1032, 2016 27576923

Arkow P: The "dark side" of the human-animal bond, in Clinician's Guide to Treating Companion Animal Issues. Edited by Kogan L, Blazina C. London, Academic Press, 2019, pp 319–346

Arluke A, Patronek G: Animal hoarding, in Animal Cruelty: A Multidisciplinary Approach to Understanding. Edited by Brewster MP, Reyes CL. Durham, NC, Carolina Academic Press, 2016, pp 199–216

Benz-Schwarzburg J, Monsó S, Huber L: How dogs perceive humans and how humans should treat their pet dogs: linking cognition with ethics. Front Psychol 11:584037, 2020 33391102

Brodie SJ, Biley FC, Shewring M: An exploration of the potential risks associated with using pet therapy in healthcare settings. J Clin Nurs 11(4):444–456, 2002 12100640

Chandler CK: Animal-Assisted Therapy in Counseling, 3rd Edition. New York, Routledge, Taylor & Francis, 2017, pp 45–71

Chur-Hansen A, McArthur M, Winefield H, et al: Animal-assisted interventions in children's hospitals: a critical review of the literature. Anthrozoos 27(1):5–18, 2014

Cieslak EJ: Animal-assisted therapy and the development of an early working alliance: the use of dogs in therapy with young adults. The University of Wisconsin-Madison, ProQuest Dissertations Publishing, 2001. Available at: www.proquest.com/docview/231305758?pq-origsite=gscholarandfromopenview=true. Accessed January 31, 2022.

Corsetti S, Ferrara M, Natoli E: Evaluating stress in dogs involved in animal-assisted interventions. Animals (Basel) 9(10):833, 2019 31635094

Custance D, Mayer J: Empathic-like responding by domestic dogs (Canis familiaris) to distress in humans: an exploratory study. Anim Cogn 15(5):851–859, 2012 22644113

Dell C, Williamson L, McKenzie H, et al: A commentary about lessons learned: transitioning a therapy dog program online during the COVID-19 pandemic. Animals (Basel) 11(3):914, 2021 33806900

Fatjó J, Bowen J, Calvo P: Stress in therapy animals, in The Welfare of Animals in Animal-Assisted Interventions: Foundations and Best Practice Methods. Edited by Peralta JM, Fine AH. Cham, Switzerland, Springer Nature, 2021, pp 91–121

Fine AH: Incorporating animal-assisted interventions into psychotherapy: guidelines and suggestions for therapists, in Handbook on Animal-Assisted Therapy: Foundations and Guidelines for Animal-Assisted Interventions, 5th Edition. Edited by Fine AH. London, Elsevier Academic Press, 2019, pp 207–224

Fine AH, Albright J, Nu J, Peralta J: Our ethical and moral responsibility: ensuring the welfare of therapy animals. Paper presented at the 2013 American Veterinary Medical Association Conference, Chicago, IL, 2013

Fine AH, Beck AM, Ng Z: The state of animal-assisted interventions: addressing the contemporary issues that will shape the future. Int J Environ Res Public Health 16(20):3997, 2019a 31635430

Fine AH, Tedeschi P, Elvove E: Forward thinking, in Handbook on Animal-Assisted Therapy: Foundations and Guidelines for Animal-Assisted Interventions, 5th Edition. Edited by Fine AH. London, Elsevier Academic Press, 2019b, pp 23–42

Finkelstein SI: Canary in a coal mine: the connection between animal abuse and human violence. Bellwether Magazine 1(58), Article 14, 2003. Available at:

https://repository.upenn.edu/bellwether/vol1/iss58/14. Accessed March 13, 2022.

Flynn E, Gandenberger J, Mueller MK, Morris KN: Animal-assisted interventions as an adjunct to therapy for youth: clinician perspectives. Child Adolesc Social Work J 37(6):631–642, 2020

Frost R: People who hoard animals. Psychiatr Times 17(4), 2000. Available at: www.psychiatrictimes.com/view/people-who-hoard-animals. Accessed November 17, 2021.

Frost RO, Steketee G, Williams L: Hoarding: a community health problem. Health Soc Care Community 8(4):229–234, 2000 11560692

Glenk LM, Kothgassner OD, Stetina BU, et al: Therapy dogs' salivary cortisol levels vary during animal-assisted interventions. Anim Welf 22(3):369–378, 2013

Hall SS, Finka L, Mills DS: A systematic scoping review: what is the risk from child-dog interactions to dog's quality of life? J Vet Behav 33:16–26, 2019

Haubenhofer DK, Kirchengast S: Physiological arousal for companion dogs working with their owners in animal-assisted activities and animal-assisted therapy. J Appl Anim Welf Sci 9(2):165–172, 2006 16956319

Haubenhofer DK, Kirchengast S: Dog handlers' and dogs' emotional and cortisol secretion responses associated with animal-assisted therapy sessions. Soc Anim 15(2):127–150, 2007

Heimlich K: Animal-assisted therapy and the severely disabled child: a quantitative study. J Rehabil 67(4):48–54, 2001

Hoarding of Animals Research Consortium: Health implications of animal hoarding. Health Soc Work 27:126–136, 2002 21608085

Horowitz A: Being a Dog: Following the Dog Into a World of Smell. New York, Scribner, 2016, pp 30–38

Huber A, Barber ALA, Faragó T, et al: Investigating emotional contagion in dogs (Canis familiaris) to emotional sounds of humans and conspecifics. Anim Cogn 20(4):703–715, 2017 28432495

Huls A: The dogs that save us. LMU Magazine, July 21, 2021. Available at: https://magazine.lmu.edu/articles/the-dogs-that-save-us. Accessed November 3, 2021.

Kaminski J, Marshall-Pescini S: The Social Dog: Behaviour and Cognition. San Diego, CA, Elsevier, 2014, pp 4–6

King C, Watters J, Mungre S: Effect of a time-out session with working animal-assisted therapy dogs. J Vet Behav 6(4):232–238, 2011

López-Cepero J: Current status of animal-assisted interventions in scientific literature: a critical comment on their internal validity. Animals (Basel) 10(6):985, 2020 32517010

MacNamara M, Moga J, Pachel C: What's love got to do with it? Selecting animals for animal-assisted mental health interventions, in Handbook on Animal-Assisted Therapy: Foundations and Guidelines for Animal-Assisted Interventions, 5th Edition. Edited by Fine AH. London, Elsevier Academic Press, 2019, pp 101–113

Maurelli MP, Santaniello A, Fioretti A, et al: The presence of *Toxocara* eggs on dog's fur as potential zoonotic risk in animal-assisted interventions: a systematic review. Animals (Basel) 9(10):827, 2019 31635019

McCullough A, Jenkins MA, Ruehrdanz A, et al: Physiological and behavioral effects of animal-assisted interventions on therapy dogs in pediatric oncology settings. Appl Anim Behav Sci 200:86–95, 2018

Meier PS, Donmall MC, McElduff P, et al: The role of the early therapeutic alliance in predicting drug treatment dropout. Drug Alcohol Depend 83(1):57–64, 2006 16298088

Melco AL, Goldman L, Fine AH, Peralta JM: Investigation of physiological and behavioral responses in dogs participating in animal-assisted therapy with children diagnosed with attention-deficit hyperactivity disorder. J Appl Anim Welf Sci 23(1):10–28, 2020 30376724

Mellor DJ, Beausoleil NJ: Extending the "Five Domains" model for animal welfare assessment to incorporate positive welfare states. Anim Welf 24(3):241–253, 2015

Mellor DJ, Patterson-Kane E, Stafford KJ: The Sciences of Animal Welfare (UFAW Animal Welfare Series). Oxford, UK, Wiley-Blackwell, 2009

Mellor DJ, Beausoleil NJ, Littlewood KE, et al: The 2020 Five Domains model: including human-animal interactions in assessments of animal welfare. Animals (Basel) 10(10):1870, 2020 33066335

Miklósi Á, Kubinyi E: Current trends in canine problem-solving and cognition. Curr Dir Psychol Sci 25(5):300–306, 2016 28503035

Miklósi A, Topál J: What does it take to become "best friends"? Evolutionary changes in canine social competence. Trends Cogn Sci 17(6):287–294, 2013 23643552

Mills DS, Dube MB, Zulch H: Stress and Pheromonatherapy in Small Animal Clinical Behaviour. Chichester, West Sussex, UK, Wiley-Blackwell, 2013, pp 4–10

Müller CA, Schmitt K, Barber AL, Huber L: Dogs can discriminate emotional expressions of human faces. Curr Biol 25(5):601–605, 2015 25683806

Murthy R, Bearman G, Brown S, et al: Animals in healthcare facilities: recommendations to minimize potential risks. Infect Control Hosp Epidemiol 36(5):495–516, 2015 25998315

Ng ZY, Fine AH: Considerations for the retirement of therapy animals. Animals (Basel) 9(12):1100, 2019 31835308

Ng ZY, Fine AH: A trajectory approach to supporting therapy animal welfare in retirement and beyond, in The Welfare of Animals in Animal-Assisted Interventions. Edited by Peralta J, Fine A. Cham, Switzerland, Springer Nature, 2021, pp 243–263

Ng ZY, Pierce BJ, Otto CM, et al: The effect of dog–human interaction on cortisol and behavior in registered animal-assisted activity dogs. Appl Anim Behav Sci 159:69–81, 2014

Ockenden EM, De Groef B, Marston L: Animal hoarding in Victoria, Australia: an exploratory study. Anthrozoos 27(1):33–47, 2014

Orlinsky DE, Ronnestad MH, Willutzki U: Fifty years of psychotherapy process-outcome research: continuity and change, in Bergin and Garfield's Handbook of Psychotherapy and Behavior Change, 5th Edition. Edited by Lambert MJ. New York, Wiley, 2003, pp 307–390

Oxley JA, Feldman MD: Complexities of maltreatment: Munchausen by proxy and animals. Companion Anim 21(10):586–589, 2016

Palagi E, Nicotra V, Cordoni G: Rapid mimicry and emotional contagion in domestic dogs. R Soc Open Sci 2(12):150505, 2015 27019737

Patronek GJ: The problem of animal hoarding. Municipal Lawyer 42(3):6–19, 2001

Patronek GJ, Nathanson JN: A theoretical perspective to inform assessment and treatment strategies for animal hoarders. Clin Psychol Rev 29(3):274–281, 2009 19254818

Patronek GJ, Loar L, Nathanson JN: Animal Hoarding: Structuring Interdisciplinary Responses to Help People, Animals and Communities at Risk. Boston, MA, Hoarding of Animals Research Consortium, 2006, pp 1–53

Peralta JM, Fine AH: The animals' perspective and its impact on welfare during animal-assisted interventions, in The Welfare of Animals in Animal-Assisted Interventions. Edited by Peralta J, Fine A. Cham, Switzerland, Springer Nature, 2021a, pp 1–20

Peralta JM, Fine AH: The welfarist and the psychologist: finding common ground in our interactions with therapy animals, in The Welfare of Animals in Animal-Assisted Interventions. Edited by Peralta J, Fine A. Cham, Switzerland, Springer Nature, 2021b, pp 265–284

Reinisch AI: Understanding the human aspects of animal hoarding. Can Vet J 49(12):1211–1214, 2008 19252714

Rooney NJ, Clark C, Casey RA: Minimizing fear and anxiety in working dogs: a review. J Vet Behav 16:53–64, 2016

Ruffman T, Morris-Trainor Z: Do dogs understand human emotional expressions? J Vet Behav 6(1):97–98, 2011

Sharf J, Primavera LH, Diener MJ: Dropout and therapeutic alliance: a meta-analysis of adult individual psychotherapy. Psychotherapy (Chic) 47(4):637–645, 2010 21198249

Svartberg K: Breed-typical behaviour in dogs—historical remnants or recent constructs? Appl Anim Behav Sci 96(3–4):293–313, 2006

Udell MA, Giglio RF, Wynne CD: Domestic dogs (Canis familiaris) use human gestures but not nonhuman tokens to find hidden food. J Comp Psychol 122(1):84–93, 2008 18298285

Uexkull JV: A stroll through the worlds of animals and men, in Instinctive Behavior. Edited by Schiller C. New York, International Universities Press, 1957, pp 5–80

VanFleet R, Fine AH, Faa-Thompson T: Application of animal-assisted interventions in professional mental health settings: an overview of practice considerations, in Handbook on Animal-Assisted Therapy: Foundations and

Guidelines for Animal-Assisted Interventions, 5th Edition. Edited by Fine AH. London, Elsevier Academic Press, 2019, pp 225–248

van Houtert EAE, Endenburg N, Rodenburg TB, Vermetten E: Do service dogs for veterans with PTSD mount a cortisol response in response to training? Animals (Basel) 11(3):650, 2021 33804470

Wanser SH, Udell MAR: Does attachment security to a human handler influence the behavior of dogs who engage in animal assisted activities? Appl Anim Behav Sci 210:88–94, 2019

Yong MH, Ruffman T: Emotional contagion: dogs and humans show a similar physiological response to human infant crying. Behav Processes 108:155–165, 2014 25452080

Roles of Animals With Individuals Who Have Mental Illness

Melissa Y. Winkle, OTR/L, FAOTA, CPDT-KA
Abigail M. Jacaruso, OTD, OTR

THE SIGNIFICANCE AND influence of animals, especially dogs, can begin very early in life as they make their appearance on children's clothing, as stuffed animals, in books, and on television, and arguably the biggest effect may come from simply having them in the home (Johnson 1996; Lobue et al. 2013; Serpell 1999; Tucker 1989). The U.S.-based American Pet Products Association (2021) estimates that the most common pet species is the dog, which is the focus of this chapter.

Relationships with dogs have been found to be meaningful across the life span (Gee and Mueller 2019). Dogs fulfill the roles of companions, emotional support animals (ESAs), and health care and human service aids for animal-assisted therapy (AAT); are facility dogs (Assistance Dogs International n.d.-a); and can be assistance dogs trained and permanently placed to serve individuals with physical, cognitive, and psychiatric disabilities (Assistance Dogs International n.d.-b). Observations of successful human-dog interactions and relationships can become quite romanticized, but many elements need to be considered to avoid disappointment and distress for the clinician, the client, and the dog. In this chapter, we provide key information to mental health providers about the health, well-being, and welfare of dogs in different roles with individuals who have mental illness and also describe some of these roles in detail.

Animal Welfare and Well-Being Considerations

Although most people are familiar with an animal's basic needs of food, water, shelter, safety, social interactions, enrichment, and veterinary care, Benz-Schwarzburg et al. (2020) describe a generalized agreement in animal ethics that humans have both negative and positive duties to animals. Negative duties refer to humans not causing harm. Positive duties refer to helping when harmful situations do occur. Mental health providers may gain insight about their clients by investigating how they treat their dogs, the relationship that clients have with their dogs, and how social situations involving others may affect the expression of the relationship (Chijiiwa et al. 2015; Nadal et al. 2020; Upadhya 2013). It can also be important to identify whether a client's pets and their associated care are a burden or a source of stress (McDonald et al. 2021). Providers may better serve their clients if they have some continuing education in the areas of humane education, basic animal husbandry, and pet loss and grief, as well as knowledge about local resources for pets.

It is critical to determine whether clients have the physical, cognitive, emotional, and financial ability to keep and care for pets, and how other household members feel about the pets. Asking clients about the number and the species of pets can provide more information about lifestyle and preferences and in some cases identify concerns such as hoarding or animal abuse. Pet dogs may also fulfill roles as ESAs, as detailed in the next section.

When clients are not able to take care of their pet(s), they can pursue a temporary foster home until they are in a better situation or seek permanent placement with another family. If a client wants a dog but is not a good candidate, volunteering at local humane associations, shelters, or rescues may be an outlet.

Knowing local animal-related ordinances and laws and ensuring that clients understand rules about pets in their housing situation can improve the quality of life for both client and dog. Bidirectional communication between the human and the dog will provide strength to their relationship. Clients should reflect on why they want or have a dog, what the dog needs and wants, and what barriers to the relationship exist. For example, if the client is continuously upset that the dog is destroying items in the home or yard and receiving complaints that the dog is barking most of the day, the client may need to determine what is causing the behavior, such as the amount of time the dog is home alone with no physical or mental stimulation. Learning about breed-specific traits may help clients understand some of the behaviors that may frustrate them and help them to identify activities to do with their pet that will improve the quality of life for both.

Health, Welfare, and Well-Being Considerations for Dogs in Any Role

Humans' relationships with dogs underwent significant evolution as humans looked to animals more for their utility, such as protecting property, sporting, entertainment, and being available on demand for human interactions. Dogs then moved from the backyard to inside our homes at the cost of asking them to refrain from normal dog behavior such as barking to communicate, licking themselves for personal hygiene, and sniffing crotches of guests to gather information. They are expected to ignore food on counters, to avoid playing with children's toys, and to be in an unattended home for several hours without relieving themselves. In almost all cases, humans believe that this is improving the dog's quality of life.

Human-animal interactions are experiencing a psychosocial metamorphosis as we develop intense relationships, and even a codependency, with companion animals. Pets offer emotional support, and therapy animals and facility dogs have become a meaningful part of our social circles. They are often included in our living situations, as pets and facility dogs are in many cases considered family (Cassels et al. 2017). Professionals are not only taking dogs to work but also asking them to participate in their jobs with AAT (Winkle and Ni 2019). Finally, as assistance dogs, they can be specifically trained to assist with tasks that humans with disabilities may not easily perform. The positive effects that dogs have on people are found in personal accounts, social media, articles, and peer-reviewed journals. However, discussions of the benefits for dogs in these positions are seen less frequently, and a dog may have a very different relationship experience, attachment style, and preferences from those of the human (Benz-Schwarzburg et al. 2020; Rehn and Keeling 2016). As the popularity of pet dogs, ESAs, facility dogs, AAT, and psychiatric service dogs grows, so should the continuing education requirement of mental health providers and their clients.

Table 3–1.   Considerations for screening clients for interactions with animals

History with animals (witnessing or participating in animal abuse, neglect, or exploitation; loss or separation from pet animal)

Developmental level, emotional intelligence, and self-management

Physical and executive functioning and sensory and psychiatric capacities

Perception of animals

Social or cultural beliefs

Experience with and interest in animals

Zoophobia and zoonosis

Allergies, immunodeficiency, respiratory disorders, and chronic compromised skin integrity

Assessment of whether animal will enhance or exacerbate the situation

Animal Assisted Intervention International (2021) has described the human-animal bond to include a mutually beneficial emotional, psychological, and physical interaction that leads to a relationship supporting the health and well-being of both humans and animals. Comparative cognition research regarding dogs' cognitive and social skills in comparison with those of humans has significantly increased in the past few decades (Benz-Schwarzburg et al. 2020). Although it is not realistic to expect all providers to specialize in both human and dog cognition, ongoing continuing education can inform some of the ethical decision-making needed to ensure the mutuality of the human-dog relationship in any role. When considering the recommendation for pets, ESAs, animal-assisted interventions, or assistance animals, providers should carefully screen client appropriateness for the interactions with an animal (Table 3–1) and ensure that the animal will be well supported (Table 3–2) (Winkle 2013).

Effect of Pets on Mental Health

Pets or companion animals are domestic animals that offer their company to us. When given the opportunity to describe relationships that matter, children have described their relationships with their pets as significant (Halldén 2003; Johnson 1996), and they may even have relationships with animals that are akin to relationships with siblings (Cassels et al. 2017; Fine et al. 2011). Bryant (1990) identified four ben-

Table 3–2. **Basic elements of dog support**

Ensure that basic needs are met	Provide food, water, shelter, safety, social interactions, enrichment, and veterinary care.
Consider the dog's perspective	How does the dog perceive their role and their experience, and do they enjoy the role and thrive in the situation?
Offer choices	Give the dog choices about if, when, and how they want to participate in their role.
Provide training	Ensure that the dog has been prepared and trained for the environment, population, and interactions.
Learn terminology	Become familiar with the terminology and learn to be realistic in your expectations of the abilities of dogs with jobs.

eficial factors of the child-pet relationship: mutuality, enduring affection, enhanced affection, and exclusivity. We would argue that this is likely true across the life span for those who enjoy dogs. Children and adolescents gain social skills from interacting with animals (Melson and Fine 2015), and those animals fulfill the four roles of attachment figures: being a source of enjoyment, providing comfort, being missed when absent, and being sought out during times of distress (Cassels et al. 2017). Young adults have been found to benefit from pets as a buffer to stress, as social capital, as coping mechanisms for mental health, and as a source of connection to identity and purpose (McDonald et al. 2021). Several studies have found that animals are beneficial to the lives of older adults as a source of companionship (Bibbo et al. 2019), for nurturance (Enders-Slegers and Hediger 2019), and for the social interactions that walking a dog provides (Curl et al. 2021).

Roles of Dogs in Mental Health Care

The nature of the interactions between dogs and owners or patients can be divided into four categories: ESAs, animal-assisted activities (AAAs), AAT, and assistance animals.

Emotional Support Animals

An ESA provides affection and support to an individual with a verifiable mental illness (Porter et al. 2021). The difference between a pet and an

ESA is that ESAs may be allowed in housing where pets are not (U.S. Department of Housing and Urban Development n.d.), and select airlines may allow ESAs to fly with their human partner at the airline's discretion (Chao 2020). According to the American Veterinary Medical Association (n.d.), the most commonly designated ESAs are dogs and cats. Although no current standards exist, there is a growing interest in ESA requests and several unscrupulous online companies that charge fees for fraudulent designation (Boness et al. 2017; Stewart et al. 2021). Companion animals, such as an ESA, may provide psychosocial benefits by helping to reduce stress or serve as a coping mechanism (McDonald et al. 2021). However, more rigorous research is needed to confirm the potential benefits (Winkle et al. 2012).

Boness et al. (2017) found that 31.4% of a sample of mental health professionals reported that they have made ESA recommendations, even though they were not familiar with the laws. The growing public and professional interest in ESAs inspired the Human-Animal Interactions in Counseling Interest Network to create a formal position paper, which recommends that counselors who lack training avoid engaging in writing letters of prescription as they may encounter potential fraud claims, such as an ESA being misrepresented as a service animal (Stewart et al. 2019).

Currently, ESA designation requires an individual to obtain formal documentation from a licensed mental health professional that the animal's presence improves the person's disability and is necessary for the individual's treatment (American Veterinary Medical Association 2017; Stewart et al. 2021). Yet few guidelines are available for documentation. Younggren et al. (2020) have proposed a model for certification of professionals conducting ESA evaluations, and Stewart et al. (2021) have made recommendations for decision-making strategies for counselors to use. Counselors should consider the needs and welfare of the client, clinic, animal, and public. Other considerations include the severity of the disability, the beneficial outcomes from having an ESA, and the appropriateness of an ESA in the individual's treatment plan (Norton 2021); also, note that a disability determination letter for an ESA may follow the client in their medical records and affect any employment security clearances (Stewart et al. 2021).

An ESA handler with a mental illness may put an animal at risk for neglect, abuse, anxiety, and injury from stressful environments and/or being handled by a person without proper training (Stewart et al. 2019). A major caution to consider with clients with mental illness seeking an ESA is that animal ownership may exacerbate existing symptoms (Stewart et al. 2021). In the event that an ESA is not the right match for a client, professionally directed AAT and incorporation of a client's relationship with their own pet, without the animal present in sessions, are alternatives to ESA designation (Stewart et al. 2021).

Because ESAs are not service animals, they do not have any public access rights (Stewart et al. 2021; U.S. Department of Justice 2015). As of December 2, 2020, airlines now recognize ESAs as pets rather than service animals, and as subject to the same policies as other pets, and travel method is subject to individual airlines' discretion (Chao 2020). The Fair Housing Act of 1988 allows appropriately documented ESAs to live in housing situations that may have no-pet policies (U.S. Department of Housing and Urban Development n.d.).

Unlike therapy and service animals, ESAs and their handlers are not required to undergo any type of formal training or evaluation (Winkle et al. 2012). Even so, the Americans With Disabilities Act has outlined handler responsibilities: 1) the animal must be under the control of the handler, 2) the animal must be housebroken, and 3) the animal must be vaccinated in accordance with local and state laws (Brennan and Nguyen 2014).

Animal-Assisted Activities

AAAs or volunteer visiting incorporates a trained and evaluated human-animal team into interactions for motivational, recreational, and social purposes and general well-being. Sessions can be goal oriented or unstructured and typically focus on social interaction, such as verbal and nonverbal interaction with the animal (Ambrosi et al. 2019; Animal Assisted Intervention International n.d.). AAAs have been found to help reduce perceived stress and associated biological markers in college students (Wood et al. 2018) and to reduce depression scores in elderly individuals (Gee and Mueller 2019). Professionals may recommend AAAs in public settings such as group homes and hospitals. Many volunteer visiting organizations provide training, evaluation, and registration for their teams.

Canines that take part in AAAs are not considered service dogs and do not have public access rights. Organizations that train and evaluate AAA animals may have standards of practice to which human-animal teams must adhere. Many of the current guidelines require that human-dog teams be reevaluated every 2–3 years and submit animal health screenings signed by a veterinarian (Serpell et al. 2020).

AAA teams undergo a minimum of introductory preparation and training (Winkle et al. 2014). Pet Partners has established criteria for prospective therapy animals that include team preparation for skills and aptitude and a course on entry-level canine body language for prospective teams. Volunteer visiting organizations have evaluators who will conduct an evaluation of the team for appropriateness of visiting.

Animal-Assisted Therapy

AAT incorporates specially trained animals into goal-directed, therapeutic intervention plans directed by health care or human service professionals (Animal Assisted Intervention International 2021). Dogs involved in AAT often help to promote improvement in different areas pertaining to a client's goals, including physical, psychosocial, cognitive, and emotional functioning, and behavior (Winkle and Ni 2019). AAT has been found to help therapists build more positive therapeutic alliances with clients, promote well-being and social functioning, and increase engagement in sessions as well as attendance in group therapy (Barak et al. 2001; Trujillo et al. 2019). The most often reported therapeutic intentions for including animals are building rapport in the therapeutic relationship and enhancing relationship skills (O'Callaghan 2008). Other professionals have reported partnering with animals in mental health treatment to model specific behaviors, encourage sharing of feelings, enhance social skills, and facilitate the feeling of a safe therapeutic environment (Chandler 2017; O'Callaghan 2008). Counselors hoping to implement AAT should undergo formal training, preparation, and supervision and adhere to the American Counseling Association's Animal-Assisted Therapy in Counseling Competencies (Stewart et al. 2016, 2021) or alternative professional international standards and competencies (Table 3–3; Winkle et al. 2022).

Clinicians should consult with their state licensing board to identify whether AAT is in their scope of practice (it may fall under alternative or complementary practices) and what the requirements are for continuing education, and they should acquire liability insurance before incorporating AAT into their practice (Winkle et al. 2014). Practitioners should gain continuing education about breed and individual traits, as well as canine communication, handling, training, health, welfare, and well-being, prior to participating (Winkle et al. 2020).

Clinicians interested in incorporating their dog into their practice can participate in intermediate to advanced training (Winkle and Ni 2019). Although many providers train and handle their own dogs, some may opt to call in an outside team from a volunteer visiting organization. Another option is for professionals to procure a professionally trained

Table 3–3. Animal Assisted Intervention International Standards of Practice for animal-assisted therapy

1. Standards for the Administration of Programs
2. Standards for the Ethical Treatment and Welfare of Participants
3. Standards for Dog Handlers and the Support of Dogs
4. Standards for the Health, Welfare, Wellbeing and Training of Dogs
5. Standards for Animal Assisted Therapy (AAT)
6. Standards for Dog Handler–Related Collaborative Animal Assisted Therapy (C-AAT)

dog from a reputable assistance dog organization, such as member organizations of Assistance Dogs International (n.d.-c). Some organizations refer to the dogs they place as *facility dogs,* and others call them *therapy dogs.* There is a debate about whether a facility dog should be considered a service dog. Service dogs serve one person with a disability, whereas dogs working in AAT serve many people with disabilities. Service dogs and dogs working in AAT may be trained in a similar manner, have similar identification and vests, and even have similar jobs (working for people with disabilities), making it difficult to tell the difference and causing debate about their public access beyond where they work. The human-animal team should be evaluated at least yearly, or when there is a change in health, environment, or population, or after a long absence from AAT (Winkle and Ni 2019). The following list includes organizations that offer international standards for AAA and AAT:

- Animal Assisted Intervention International (2021): https://aai-int.org
- International Association of Human-Animal Interaction Organizations (2018): https://iahaio.org
- Society for Companion Animal Studies (2019): www.scas.org.uk

Assistance Animals

The three categories of assistance dogs are guide, hearing, and service. Service dogs are trained to perform a wide variety of tasks for individuals with disabilities other than deafness or blindness (Assistance Dogs International n.d.-a). For the purpose of this chapter, only psychiatric service dogs are explored.

Psychiatric service dogs differ from ESAs because service dogs perform trained tasks (U.S. Department of Justice 2015) to aid an individual with a psychiatric disorder, including but not limited to PTSD, bipolar disorder, schizophrenia, anxiety, depression, and panic disorder (Esnayra and Love 2008; Lloyd et al. 2019). A study by Lloyd et al. (2019) found that service dogs may reduce suicide attempts and hospitalizations and increase confidence in attending appointments.

Service dogs have the potential to improve the quality of life and independence of an individual living with a mental illness. Mental health providers are often responsible for the documentation to support a service dog, requiring these providers to evaluate client needs and understand what service dogs are realistically capable of doing (Porter et al. 2021). Providers also should have knowledge of service dog laws and the individual service dog training organization requirements for placement of dogs.

Assistance Dogs International is a coalition of nonprofit organizations that raise, train, and place different types of assistance dogs. Selecting a dog from an Assistance Dogs International Accredited Member program ensures that an individual is receiving an assistance dog from a program that is meeting the highest standards in the industry and that the service dog handler will also be educated (Assistance Dogs International n.d.-b). Most service dog organizations will require the individual to complete an application, which includes providing their diagnoses and a professional evaluation of how a service dog may improve their disability status. This process can be rather burdensome for the health care provider and requires knowledge of what service dogs can do for individuals with specific disabilities and review of the limited research on benefits of service dog partnerships. Providers should be aware of the potential for a service dog to exacerbate mental health conditions or for individuals to experience decreased mental health after acquiring a service dog (Stewart et al. 2021; Yamamoto and Hart 2019).

Psychiatric service dogs are trained to perform a variety of tasks to assist an individual with a mental illness, such as grounding to help reduce anxiety, nudging or pawing to bring back awareness, establishing body contact to reduce anxiety, providing deep pressure stimulation, blocking others from coming too close to their owner, comforting the individual on waking from night terrors, and interrupting episodes of anger (Lloyd et al. 2019). A service dog may also be trained to assist their handler in leaving a situation and finding an exit if the handler is experiencing social anxiety (Yamamoto and Hart 2019), or a service dog may be trained to alert to real noises or people, to differentiate from hallucinations experienced by a handler. Professionally trained service dogs are traditionally trained for obedience and for public access, and the training is tailored to the unique needs of the human they will assist. In the United States, people with psychiatric disabilities who partner with service dogs are afforded all of the rights that other assistance dog partners have (Table 3–4). Regulations and laws regarding assistance dogs vary among cities, states, and countries, and it is recommended that providers and clients investigate their regional laws (Bremhorst et al. 2018).

Key Clinical Points

- Mental health providers should have an understanding of fundamental information on current terminology, definitions and descriptions, roles of the clinician, client screening, preparation of dogs, and laws and guidelines related to several jobs that dogs do under the mental health umbrella.

- Mental health providers have a professional obligation to seek out additional continuing education related to assistance animals and stay current on changes to laws and regulations that affect their participation in emotional support animal and psychiatric service dog recommendations, referrals, and documentation.

- Mental health providers should consider the meaningfulness and motivation that dogs may provide in various roles but also keep in mind that not every client who likes dogs would benefit from working with them.

- Consideration must be given to the dogs in our clients' lives to ensure that they experience the best health, welfare, and well-being we can offer.

References

Ambrosi C, Zaiontz C, Peragine G, et al: Randomized controlled study on the effectiveness of animal-assisted therapy on depression, anxiety, and illness perception in institutionalized elderly. Psychogeriatrics 19(1):55–64, 2019 30221438

American Pet Products Association: Pet industry market size, trends & ownership statistics. 2021. Available at: https://www.americanpetproducts.org/press_industrytrends.asp. Accessed December 16, 2021.

Table 3–4. Public access laws in the United States

Law	Description	Website
Americans With Disabilities Act (ADA)	Allows service dogs and handlers in public facilities and accommodations.	https://adata.org/guide/service-animals-and-emotional-support-animals
U.S. Department of Transportation (DOT) Service Animal Final Ruling: *Traveling by Air With Service Animals*	December 10, 2020, ruling that requires passengers with service animals to complete U.S. DOT Service Animal Form and the Service Animal Relief Attestation. Recognizes emotional support animals as pets and not as service animals.	www.transportation.gov/sites/dot.gov/files/2020-12/Final%20Service%20Animal%20Rule%20%28FR%20Version%29.pdf
U.S. Department of Housing and Urban Development	Protects individuals with service dogs in obtaining housing and reasonable accommodations, such as the waiver of pet deposit fee or ability to live at a property that has a no-pet policy.	www.hud.gov/program_offices/fair_housing_equal_opp/assistance_animals
Public Access Laws United States (Assistance Dogs International)	Identifies resources on public access laws in the United States	https://assistancedogsinternational.org/resources/public-access-laws-united-states

American Veterinary Medical Association: Assistance Animals: Rights of Access and the Problem of Fraud. 2017. Available at: https://www.avma.org/sites/default/files/resources/Assistance-Animals-Rights-Access-Fraud-AVMA.pdf. Accessed December 5, 2021.

American Veterinary Medical Association: Emotional support animals. n.d. Available at: https://www.avma.org/resources-tools/avma-policies/emotional-support-animals. Accessed December 16, 2021.

Animal Assisted Intervention International: Animal Assisted Therapy: Standards, Accreditation Processes and Manual, Glossary and General Competencies. 2021. Available at: https://aai-int.org/wp-content/uploads/2021/04/AAT-Public-Booklet-Watermark-21-February-2021.pdf. Accessed December 5, 2021.

Animal Assisted Intervention International: Glossary of terms. n.d. Available at: https://aai-int.org/aai/glossary-of-terms. Accessed December 6, 2021.

Assistance Dogs International: ADI terms and definitions. n.d.-a. Available at: https://assistancedogsinternational.org/resources/adi-terms-definitions. Accessed December 16, 2021.

Assistance Dogs International: Looking for an assistance dog. n.d.-b. Available at: https://assistancedogsinternational.org/main/looking-for-an-assistance-dog. Accessed December 16, 2021.

Assistance Dogs International: Member search. n.d.-c. Available at: https://assistancedogsinternational.org/resources/member-search. Accessed December 16, 2021.

Barak Y, Savorai O, Mavashev S, Beni A: Animal-assisted therapy for elderly schizophrenic patients: a one-year controlled trial. Am J Geriatr Psychiatry 9(4):439–442, 2001 11739071

Benz-Schwarzburg J, Monsó S, Huber L: How dogs perceive humans and how humans should treat their pet dogs: linking cognition with ethics. Front Psychol 11:584037, 2020 33391102

Bibbo J, Curl AL, Johnson RA: Pets in the lives of older adults: a life course perspective. Anthrozoos 32(4):541–554, 2019

Boness CL, Younggren JN, Frumkin IB: The certification of emotional support animals: differences between clinical and forensic mental health practitioners. Prof Psychol Res Pr 48(3):216–223, 2017

Bremhorst A, Mongillo P, Howell T, Marinelli L: Spotlight on assistance dogs—legislation, welfare and research. Animals (Basel) 8(8):129, 2018 30049995

Brennan J, Nguyen V: Service animals and emotional support animals: where are they allowed and under what conditions? ADA National Network, 2014. Available at: https://adata.org/guide/service-animals-and-emotional-support-animals. Accessed December 5, 2021.

Bryant BK: The richness of the child-pet relationship: a consideration of both benefits and costs of pets to children. Anthrozoos 3(4):253–261, 1990

Cassels MT, White N, Gee N, Hughes C: One of the family? Measuring young adolescents' relationships with pets and siblings. J Appl Dev Psychol 49:12–20, 2017

Chandler CK: Animal-Assisted Therapy in Counseling, 3rd Edition. New York, Routledge, 2017

Chao E: Traveling by Air With Service Animals. U.S. Department of Transportation, 14 CFR Part 382, November 30, 2020. Available at: https://www.transportation.gov/sites/dot.gov/files/2020-12/Service%20Animal%20Final%20Rule.pdf. Accessed December 5, 2021.

Chijiiwa H, Kuroshima H, Hori Y, et al: Dogs avoid people who behave negatively to their owner: third-party affective evaluation. Anim Behav 106:123–127, 2015

Curl AL, Bibbo J, Johnson RA: Neighborhood engagement, dogs, and life satisfaction in older adulthood. J Appl Gerontol 40(12):1706–1714, 2021

Enders-Slegers MJ, Hediger K: Pet ownership and human–animal interaction in an aging population: rewards and challenges. Anthrozoos 32(2):255–265, 2019

Esnayra J, Love C: A survey of mental health patients utilizing psychiatric service dogs. January 2008. Available at: https://www.researchgate.net/publication/265102711_A_Survey_of_Mental_Health_Patients_Utilizing_Psychiatric_Service_Dogs. Accessed March 27, 2022.

Fine AH, Dennis AL, Bowers C: Incorporating animal-assisted interventions in therapy with boys at risk, in Engaging Boys in Treatment. Edited by Haen C. New York, Routledge, 2011, pp 137–156

Gee NR, Mueller MK: A systematic review of research on pet ownership and animal interactions among older adults. Anthrozoos 32(2):183–207, 2019

Halldén G: Children's views of family, home and house, in Children in the City: Home, Neighbourhood and Community. Edited by Christensen P, O'Brien M. London, RoutledgeFalmer, 2003, pp 29–45

International Association of Human-Animal Interaction Organizations: IAHAIO White Paper: The IAHAIO definitions for animal assisted intervention and guidelines for wellness of animals involved in AAI. 2018. Available at: https://iahaio.org/wp/wp-content/uploads/2021/01/iahaio-white-paper-2018-english.pdf. Accessed December 5, 2021.

Johnson KR: The ambiguous terrain of petkeeping in children's realistic animal stories. Soc Anim 4(1):1–17, 1996

Lloyd J, Johnston L, Lewis J: Psychiatric assistance dog use for people living with mental health disorders. Front Vet Sci 6:166, 2019 31245389

Lobue V, Bloom Pickard M, Sherman K, et al: Young children's interest in live animals. Br J Dev Psychol 31(Pt 1):57–69, 2013 23331106

McDonald SE, Matijczak A, Nicotera N, et al: "He was like, my ride or die": sexual and gender minority emerging adults' perspectives on living with pets during the transition to adulthood. Emerg Adulthood 10(4):1008–1025, 2021. Available at: https://journals.sagepub.com/doi/abs/10.1177/21676968211025340#. Accessed December 5, 2021.

Melson GF, Fine AH: Animals in the lives of children, in Handbook on Animal-Assisted Therapy, 4th Edition. Edited by Fine AH. San Diego, CA, Academic Press, 2015, pp 179–194

Nadal Z, Ferrari M, Lora J, et al: Noah's syndrome: systematic review of animal hoarding disorder. Hum Anim Interact Bull 10(1):1–21, 2020

Norton AL: Political ideologies, political party affiliation, and treatment decisions of clinical mental health counselors. Ph.D. Dissertation, University of South Florida, 2021. Available at: https://digitalcommons.usf.edu/etd/8835. Accessed December 16, 2021.

O'Callaghan DM: Exploratory study of animal assisted therapy interventions used by mental health professionals. University of North Texas, ProQuest Dissertations Publishing, May 2008. Available at: https://www.proquest.com/openview/ce774c0fb2af579f518446120db846f5/1?pq-origsite=gscholarandcbl=18750. Accessed December 16, 2021.

Porter M, Winkle MY, Herlache-Pretzer E: Considerations for recommending service dogs versus emotional support animals for veterans with post-traumatic stress disorder. People Anim 4(1):4, 2021. Available at: https://docs.lib.purdue.edu/paij/vol4/iss1/4. Accessed December 5, 2021.

Rehn T, Keeling LJ: Measuring dog-owner relationships: crossing boundaries between animal behaviour and human psychology. Appl Anim Behav Sci 183:1–9, 2016

Serpell J: Guest editor's introduction: animals in children's lives. Soc Anim 7(2):87–94, 1999

Serpell JA, Kruger KA, Freeman LM, et al: Current standards and practices within the therapy dog industry: results of a representative survey of United States therapy dog organizations. Front Vet Sci 7:35, 2020 32118059

Society for Companion Animal Studies: Animal Assisted Interventions: SCAS Code of Practice for the UK. 2019. Available at: http://www.scas.org.uk/wp-content/uploads/2019/08/SCAS-AAI-Code-of-Practice-August-2019.pdf. Accessed December 5, 2021.

Stewart LA, Chang CY, Parker LK, Grubbs N: Animal-Assisted Therapy in Counseling Competencies. Alexandria, VA, American Counseling Association, Animal-Assisted Therapy in Mental Health Interest Network, 2016. Available at: https://www.counseling.org/docs/default-source/competencies/animal-assisted-therapy-competencies-june-2016.pdf. Accessed December 16, 2021.

Stewart L, Johnson A, Taylor C, et al: Emotional support animals: Human Animal Interventions in Counseling Interest Network position statement. American Counseling Association, 2019. Available at: https://www.unh.edu/sites/default/files/departments/student_accessibility_services_/aca.final_version_esa14556_002.pdf. Accessed December 6, 2021.

Stewart LA, Hakenewerth TJ, Rabinowitz P, Fowler H: Using holistic and ethical practices with emotional support animal requests. J Creat Ment Health April 26, 2021. Available at: https://doi.org/10.1080/15401383.2021.1911723. Accessed December 5, 2021.

Trujillo KC, Kuo GT, Hull ML, et al: Engaging adolescents: animal assisted therapy for adolescents with psychiatric and substance use disorders. J Child Fam Stud 29(2):307–314, 2019

Tucker N: Animals in children's literature, in The Status of Animals: Ethics, Education and Welfare. Edited by Paterson D, Palmer M. Wallingford, UK, Oxford University Press, 1989, pp 167–172

Upadhya V: The abuse of animals as a method of domestic violence: the need for criminalization. Emory Law J 63:1163–1210, 2013

U.S. Department of Housing and Urban Development: Assistance animals. n.d. Available at: https://www.hud.gov/program_offices/fair_housing_equal_opp/assistance_animals. Accessed December 16, 2021.

U.S. Department of Justice: Frequently asked questions about service animals and the ADA. July 2015. Available at: https://www.ada.gov/regs2010/service_animal_qa.html. Accessed December 16, 2021.

Winkle MY: Professional Applications of Animal Assisted Interventions: Blue Dog Book, 2nd Edition. Albuquerque, NM, Dogwood Therapy Services, 2013

Winkle MY, Ni K: Animal assisted occupational therapy: guidelines for standards, theory, and practice, in Handbook on Animal-Assisted Therapy: Foundations and Guidelines for Animal-Assisted Interventions, 5th Edition. Edited by Fine AH. London, Elsevier Academic Press, 2019, pp 381–395

Winkle M, Crowe TK, Hendrix I: Service dogs and people with physical disabilities partnerships: a systematic review. Occup Ther Int 19(1):54–66, 2012 21858889

Winkle MY, Wilder A, Jackson LZ: Dogs as pets, visitors, therapists and assistants. Home Healthc Nurse 32(10):589–595, 2014 25370974

Winkle M, Johnson A, Mills D: Dog welfare, well-being and behavior: considerations for selection, evaluation and suitability for animal-assisted therapy. Animals (Basel) 10(11):2188, 2020 33238376

Winkle M, Rogers J, Gorbing P, Vancoppernolle D: Animal Assisted Intervention International Public Document: Standards of Practice and Competencies for Animal Assisted Interventions. 2022. Available at: https://aai-int.org/wp-content/uploads/2022/07/AAII-Standards-and-Comp-June-24-2022-.pdf. Accessed August 18, 2022.

Wood E, Ohlsen S, Thompson J, et al: The feasibility of brief dog-assisted therapy on university students stress levels: the PAwS study. J Ment Health 27(3):263–268, 2018 28984144

Yamamoto M, Hart LA: Providing guidance on psychiatric service dogs and emotional support animals, in Clinician's Guide to Treating Companion Animal Issues. Edited by Kogan L, Blazina C. London, Academic Press, 2019, pp 77–101

Younggren JN, Boness CL, Bryant LM, Koocher GP: Emotional support animal assessments: toward a standard and comprehensive model for mental health professionals. Prof Psychol Res Pr 51(2):156–162, 2020 32982035

4

Companion Animals in Crisis Intervention

Leslie Stewart, Ph.D., LCPC, C-AAIS
Jennifer Hightower, Ph.D., NCC

ACCORDING TO Gerald Caplan (1964), a *crisis* is an obstacle that is temporarily insurmountable through an individual's typical methods of problem-solving. Kleepsies (2014) expanded on Caplan's (1964) definition and described a crisis as a brief episode of intense emotional distress during which an individual's usual coping methods do not provide relief or improve functioning. This means that during a crisis, an individual's perceived coping resources are not sufficient to meet their current perceived environmental demands (Lazarus and Folkman 1984). The discrepancy between perceived coping resources and perceived environmental demands can present a double-edged sword for the individual in crisis. On one hand, it offers a heightened potential for growth and increased resilience in future crisis events. At the same time, an individual can experience further deterioration of coping skills and increased vulnerability to future stressors. Because crisis involves the subjective relationship between each person's perceived coping resources and perceived environmental demands, the actual cause of a crisis episode may vary widely, as can effective crisis resolutions (France 2014). A situation that is navigable for one person may constitute a crisis for another. Crises may be individual or large-scale in nature and may be human caused or environmentally caused. However, all crises share five essential characteristics that are agreed on by crisis researchers (e.g., Caplan 1964; France 2014) (Table 4–1).

Crisis will affect every person, community, and system, often multiple times during a lifetime. Across age groups, nationalities, and cultures, crisis is one of the great human universalizers. Even though it is a normal human experience, crisis feels painful, chaotic, paralyzing, and terrifying, and it seems far outside of our personal perception of normal. The frequency and prevalence of crisis creates an ever-growing need for well-trained crisis responders who are able to competently implement innovative and efficient strategies for helping those in crisis.

Clinical Presentation and Longitudinal Time Course

Although the experience of crisis may be universal, the discipline of crisis response is highly specific. Ethical and effective crisis responders use foundational anthropological and neurobiological knowledge about the human stress response to plan strategic interventions at each stage of crisis that are tailored to assist in each unique situation. Crisis causes and outcomes vary unpredictably, but the human stress response remains fairly consistent across most types of crisis in most individuals. Crisis-affected individuals often experience memory failures and difficulties in problem-solving and decision-making, as well as difficulty regulating intense emotions such as fear, anger, hostility, grief, hopelessness, helplessness, and a sense of alienation or isolation from others (Briere and Scott 2014). This temporary impairment means that many crisis-affected individuals are not able to cope with the crisis situation in the same way as they cope with other stressors and may require support from crisis responders, mental health and first-response professionals, and loved ones (Briere and Scott 2014).

Of particular importance is differentiating between crisis and trauma. Crisis and trauma are both considered to be personal and subjective rather than defined by objective external events. Both experiences are considered to be universal human experiences, and both involve similar activation of the human stress response. Although the two experiences share several key commonalities, they are categorized separately and require different intervention approaches for treatment.

One important difference is the time frame for resolution. As stated earlier, a key characteristic of a crisis is that it is a time-limited experience and is usually resolved, for better or worse, within a period of approx-

Table 4-1. Essential characteristics of crisis

Characteristic of crisis	Description
Precipitated by a specific event	Identifiable event: perceived environmental demands greatly outweighing perceived coping resources; can be single distressing event or cumulative experiences
Inevitable	Part of human condition: all people or systems will encounter crises
Personal and subjective	Perception of event more important than objective occurrence; defined by discrepancy between perceived coping resources and perceived environmental demands rather than by event
Resolution in brief period of time	Differentiated from trauma, which lasts for extended amounts of time
Adaptive or maladaptive resolution	End or resolution can take many forms, including combination of adaptive and maladaptive

Source.   Based on Caplan 1964; France 2014.

imately 2 months (France 2014). According to Briere and Scott (2014), many traumas may begin as a crisis event, but the length of time to resolve the experience becomes prolonged past the approximate 2-month time frame. Another key difference between crisis and trauma is the relationship between perceived coping resources and perceived environmental demands. In crisis, an individual experiences a discrepancy between perceived coping resources and perceived environmental demands. In trauma, this discrepancy is even greater and is accompanied by a destruction of personal meaning or disruption of an individual's functioning (Briere and Scott 2014). Therefore, effective crisis response aims to reduce the discrepancy between perceived environmental demands and perceived coping resources immediately and in the short term, while effective trauma interventions involve settling the long-term discrepancy between perceived environmental demands and perceived coping resources and include repair work and reconstruction of the individual's personal meaning and functioning (Briere and Scott 2014). The primary goal of crisis intervention is to prevent further deterioration of coping while working to return to precrisis functioning. Effective crisis response stabilizes the affected individual to maximize the potential for the crisis to be a resilience-fostering experience rather than an experience that results in increased vulnerability to future stressors (France 2014). Effective crisis response involves the use of strong interpersonal skills and a basic knowledge of the human stress response, but it is not considered to be counseling or psychotherapy.

Overview of Existing Evidence-Based Treatments

Many theories and models of crisis intervention exist, but the most effective strategies are those that are flexible, relationally engaging, and informed by the unique neurobiology of the brain in crisis (Siegel 2010). One such strategy is animal-assisted crisis response (AACR). In order to fully appreciate and conceptualize this highly specialized and nuanced approach, one must first understand foundational concepts of general crisis and crisis response.

Most volunteer responders will encounter individuals during what is referred to as the *impact stage*. In this stage, affected individuals are experiencing an initial response to a crisis (France 2014). Normal responses in this stage include helplessness, anxiety, agitated depression, anger, and social withdrawal. During this stage, survivors need immediate anxiety relief and contact and engagement with calm and stable others to help regulate the fight/flight/freeze response and to ease feelings of alienation, isolation, and helplessness. Establishing contact and engagement can be particularly challenging during the impact stage, because the person may appear highly emotionally distressed or unresponsive. Effective support during this stage aims to provide comfort and safety. Toward this end, an effective response must appear stable, supportive, and structured. Responders use active listening skills and empathy to connect with survivors and may occasionally need creative strategies to gain the survivor's attention, direct the survivor to assistance resources, or encourage the survivor to move away from dangerous environmental conditions (France 2014). At the impact stage, simply providing a calm, validating, and stable presence without trying to change the survivor's feelings is a highly effective and consistent intervention strategy (France 2014).

Animal-Assisted Crisis Response

AACR is a highly specialized application of animal-assisted activities, wherein highly trained and evaluated volunteer human-animal teams assist crisis responders to support the psychological and physiological needs of individuals affected by and responding to crises and disasters in complex, unpredictable environments (Pet Partners 2019). It is important for readers to recognize that although equally valuable, AACR is considered a form of animal-assisted activity, which differs in boundaries, scope, and delivery from the animal-assisted therapy provided by licensed mental health providers during counseling or psychotherapy for individuals experiencing symptoms of trauma. Although AACR teams are trained in foundational principles of crisis response, they themselves are not considered to be crisis responders (Greenbaum 2006). The role of an AACR handler and the role of a professional crisis responder are mutually exclusive, even if the handler is qualified to serve as a crisis response mental health professional (Greenbaum 2006). For the well-being of all humans and animals involved, crisis responders must not simultaneously perform both the role of professional crisis responder and the role of crisis response mental health professional (Lackey and Haberstock 2019). Rather, the AACR handler seeks to connect the survivor with a crisis responder after facilitating the human-animal interaction. In AACR, the human handler's primary focus is on the animal and facilitating safe, engaging, and mutually beneficial human-animal interactions with survivors, grounded in the knowledge of the unique, species-specific ethology of their animal partners (International Institute for Animal Assisted Play Therapy 2022). By contrast, the crisis responder's primary focus is on the human survivor. This differentiation may be an adjustment for some providers of animal-assisted therapy or animal-assisted education who simultaneously serve as the animal handler and the human service provider in predictable professional environments. In short, AACR requires in-depth and extensive training and preparation for the human and animal involved but is differentiated from professional health care, professional mental health treatment, and professional crisis response (Greenbaum 2006).

The first documented inclusion of specially trained dog/handler teams in crisis response occurred in 1995 when the Federal Emergency Management Agency (FEMA) requested the presence of therapy dog/handler teams in the aftermath of the Murrah Federal Building bombings in Oklahoma (Lackey and Haberstock 2019; Shubert 2012). Since then, specially trained animal/handler teams have been invited to assist crisis responders in numerous natural disasters and episodes of mass violence (Greenbaum 2006; Lackey and Haberstock 2019). In response to the growing need for teams to assist in disasters while simultaneously protecting animal welfare and ensuring appropriateness of participation, Cindy Ehlers founded Hope Animal-Assisted Crisis Response

(HOPE AACR) in 1998 (Lackey and Haberstock 2019; National Standards Committee for Animal-Assisted Crisis Response 2010). HOPE AACR is credited with formalizing AACR and setting a precedent for the specialized and formal training necessary for safe and ethical implementation of this response (Lackey and Haberstock 2019). The empirical literature specific to the formalized application of current AACR is in its infancy, although anecdotal observations of AACR's unique effect on the crisis response process are represented in the conceptual and theoretical literature. In selected articles (Bua 2013; Chandler 2008; Lackey and Haberstock 2019; National Standards Committee for Animal-Assisted Crisis Response 2010; Shubert 2012), several common themes emerge: 1) AACR teams engage withdrawn, isolated, or unresponsive survivors more effectively than do human-only responders; 2) AACR teams assist survivors in grounding and anxiety reduction quickly; 3) dogs involved in AACR are perceived to help identify individuals who need the most support from crisis responders; and 4) AACR teams are heavily sought out by crisis responders for their own stress. These themes are consistent with existing empirical findings for competently implemented animal-assisted interventions (AAIs) in general. Below, we view the application of AACR through the lens of specific supportive strategies associated with the impact stage of a crisis.

Contact and Engagement

During a crisis, many individuals naturally isolate, withdraw, and become unresponsive. This can present a unique challenge to a crisis responder, who is tasked with engaging survivors in order to facilitate movement toward resources and recovery. Particularly in the impact stage of a crisis, many human crisis responders experience difficulty establishing psychological and verbal contact with isolated and withdrawn survivors. AACR teams may assist in this process through one of the most frequently touted benefits of all AAIs: the unique effect on rapport building (Chandler 2017).

Positive human-animal interactions are associated with increased oxytocin (Chandler 2017) and decreased cortisol (Siegel 2010) levels. When oxytocin increases and cortisol decreases, humans experience calmness, decreased depression, decreased heart rate and blood pressure, and increased trust and social skills (Siegel 2010). By engaging a survivor in interactions with the animal, the AACR team may help the crisis responder engage the survivor more quickly and effectively, while simultaneously providing opportunities for the survivor's brain and body to calm. It is important to note that the AACR team should approach the survivor only when given a clear indication, verbally or nonverbally, that the survivor wants to interact with the animal. Inexperienced or overly enthusiastic AACR teams may inadvertently cause further withdrawal if the animal's approach is unwanted or perceived as intrusive by the survivor.

Safety and Comfort

After establishing contact with the survivor, the next task of a crisis responder is to provide a sense of safety and comfort for the survivor. The provision of safety and comfort must happen before the survivor is able to regulate their physiological, emotional, and cognitive responses. In addition to the potential comfort a survivor may experience through interacting with and touching the animal, AACR may provide the survivor with nonverbal avenues for expression and communication, because accessing verbal language may be difficult during a crisis (Greenbaum 2006). The trust and social bonding boost offered by the AACR team may also increase the likelihood that the survivor will trust and relate to the handler. Humans handling friendly and healthy animals are often perceived by survivors as more trustworthy than a human without an animal (Lackey and Haberstock 2019), potentially making it easier to motivate a survivor to move away from danger or toward another resource.

State Anxiety Management and Grounding

As discussed earlier, most animal-assisted activities, including AACR, are intended to help address immediate experiences of stress and anxiety happening in the here and now. This is particularly applicable to the conduct of AACR during the impact stage of a crisis, when survivors are experiencing an increase in stress-related physiological, cognitive, and emotional symptoms. Symptoms of crisis stress responses often include elevated heart rate, high blood pressure, and increased cortisol levels, as well as a sense of detachment, disorientation, numbness, racing thoughts, and distortion of time and space (Lackey and Haberstock 2019). Provided that the survivor's interaction with an AACR team is positive and voluntary, AACR may provide relief from some immediate physiological and psychological fight/flight/freeze responses. Studies conducted by multiple authors (Bua 2013; Shiloh et al. 2003) indicate that for many individuals, positive human-animal interactions, such as interacting with, touching, talking to, and observing calm and friendly animals, significantly decrease all of the crisis-related stress symptoms described earlier. Furthermore, van der Kolk (2014) articulated that connection to the five senses and grounding in the present moment are also necessary to regulate distressing emotions so that the survivor can think more clearly and access assistance. According to Lackey and Haberstock (2019), for individuals who are comfortable with dogs, the presence of a dog engages all five senses comfortably and nonintrusively. When these specific crisis-related symptoms and concerns are adequately addressed, survivors may be better able to access areas of the brain needed for planning, problem-solving, and short-term resilience.

Connection With Crisis Responders and Resources

Possibly the most important task of an AACR team is to facilitate connection and communication between the survivor and the professional first responders. Through the unique effect of human-animal interactions, AACR can facilitate that connection more quickly and with greater ease than many other crisis intervention strategies. By establishing connection and increasing trust, an AACR handler can encourage and empower the survivor to identify and seek much needed support. For example, an AACR team might escort a survivor to on-site professional medical providers for essential treatment. In some cases, professional first responders may even ask an AACR team to stay with the survivor if they are fearful or nervous about receiving medical attention or other support. Although this is one of many valuable ways that AACR teams may support survivors, it is important to follow the first responder's instructions about this level of involvement and accompaniment. Effective AACR teams are careful not to interrupt, impede, or otherwise interfere with first responder tasks.

AACR teams also provide much-needed support to the first responders, medical professionals, and mental health professionals who are affected by the demands of professional crisis response (Greenbaum 2006). Exhaustion resulting from this work affects all areas of responders' well-being, including physical, emotional, and mental wellness (Figley 1995). Crisis first responders are often affected by vicarious trauma and experience many of the same physiological, cognitive, and emotional symptoms present in survivors. Thus, interventions that benefit crisis survivors, such as AACR, also benefit first responders in ways similar to those already described. It is recommended that AACR teams make themselves available to support first responders in addition to the survivors themselves.

Animal-Assisted Crisis Response Teams and Vicarious Trauma

Human handlers of AACR teams are also vulnerable to burnout and vicarious trauma. Because they support affected individuals and crisis first responders, it is particularly important for AACR handlers to be aware of the potential effect of burnout and vicarious trauma on their own well-being. Like many crisis responders, AACR teams work in overwhelming conditions, and though they may not be experiencing the crisis themselves, they risk burnout and vicarious trauma by engaging in emotionally taxing work over an extended period of time. AACR handlers experiencing burnout may show exhaustion, fatigue, lack of motivation, loss of satisfaction, detachment, dehumanization, depression, feelings of inadequacy, and a decline in physical or mental health. Vicarious trauma responses may include maladaptive coping, chronic stress response, diminished sense of meaning, interpersonal and identity disruptions, and increased risk for suicidality and self-harm. Certain symptoms associated with this experience, such as detachment and impaired empathy, can make attending to the welfare of an animal partner more difficult. AACR handlers have an ethical responsibility to self-monitor and address any emerging impairments or signs of burnout. Although HOPE AACR and Pet Partners AACR handler training covers burnout and vicarious trauma prevention, we recommend that AACR handlers proactively create a wellness plan for themselves and their animal partner before engaging in crisis work, and they should seek professional mental health services if they notice symptoms of vicarious trauma in themselves.

Ethics and Best Practices

The unique potential benefits associated with appropriately facilitated AACR make it an attractive option for supporting individuals affected by crisis. However, handlers must be prepared to address the unique ethical considerations of working with animals in complex and unpredictable environments. AACR handlers are responsible for seamlessly and consistently safeguarding animal and human welfare in highly unpredictable, complex, and potentially even dangerous or volatile environments. Because of the complexity of these additional demands, AACR teams require training and evaluation beyond those provided in the general registration categories offered by many therapy animal registration organizations. Most AACR organizations require experience as a registered animal/handler team, but traditional registration as an AAI team is not sufficient to qualify for AACR suitability (Pet Partners 2019). Furthermore, not all animals appropriate for general AAIs are also appropriate for AACR. According to Chandler (2017), therapy animals should not be brought to crisis situations unless they have been evaluated for exceptionally high tolerance for stress, chaos, and noise; consistently respond to handler cues in the presence of distractions; and are highly sociable in almost all environments toward almost all people. For example, one of the authors currently works with three animal partners, all of which are suitable for and well adapted to animal-assisted therapy and animal-assisted education in a predictable university setting. Of all three highly sociable, reliable, and experienced animal partners, none would be comfortable in chaotic disaster situations, even with attentive handler support. Similarly, not all AAI human handlers are appropriate for AACR. AACR handlers must be experienced, tolerant of chaotic and stressful situations, knowledgeable about crisis response, and emotionally and psychologically stable; they also must have shown a consistent ability to effectively attend to and advocate for animal welfare in all situations. Handlers who are currently navigating their own crisis situations or mental health concerns should pause their AACR availability until those concerns are appropriately addressed.

Clinical and Animal Welfare Considerations

Because of the intense and unpredictable nature of crisis situations, AACR handlers must be aware of the welfare and well-being implications for affected individuals and for their animal partners. As discussed earlier in this chapter, many well-intentioned attempts to provide comfort during crisis situations may inadvertently cause harm. For this reason, ethical AACR handlers are mindful of their scope of practice and avoid attempting to provide short-term counseling or psychotherapy during crisis situations. Additionally, it is essential that handlers avoid offering advice, problem-solving, anecdotes, silver-lining explanations, or unsolicited spiritual guidance, because such responses may be trivializing, frightening, or offensive to the survivor. Ethical responders avoid making false promises or reassurances (e.g., "Everything will be alright"), guaranteeing availability of resources, or offering false hope. To best avoid harm, handlers must remain mindful of the boundaries of their role in facilitating connections between survivors and crisis responders.

All ethical AAIs involve a heavy emphasis on maintaining the animal's safety, comfort, and well-being. In AACR, animals may face additional risks and require additional handler support. Safety conditions associated with crisis situations must be thoroughly assessed before involving an animal. Temperature, air quality, biohazards, crowding, and debris could present physical safety concerns. In addition, AACR animals will likely face intense human emotions, including potential emotional distress from the handler, which can be overwhelming and potentially frightening for many animals. Given that most crisis conditions exacerbate stress and fatigue in even the most prepared AACR animals, handlers must gather as much information as possible about the crisis situation and environment before arriving with their animal partner, create a proactive animal advocacy plan specific to the situation and individual animal's needs, and comply with the 2-hour maximum visit time established by Pet Partners AACR. As discussed earlier, handlers also should be aware of the potential for their own burnout or vicarious trauma symptoms to affect their ability to effectively support and advocate for their animal partner.

Credentialing and National Standards

Although some professional associations such as the American Counseling Association (Stewart et al. 2016) have formalized AAI provider competencies and industry leaders such as Pet Partners (2018) and Animal Assisted Intervention International (n.d.) have highly specific standards of practice for AAIs, there is no current legal or governmental oversight of AAIs in general. This lack of oversight and regulation makes AACR specialty certifications critically important as indicators that a human-animal team is appropriately prepared to navigate the complex and highly nuanced ethical best practices associated with AACR. Psychiatrists seeking appropriately qualified AACR teams should look for industry-leading AACR registration such as HOPE AACR and Pet Partners AACR as a minimum standard for potential inclusion.

In 2010, HOPE AACR and NATIONAL Crisis Response Canines collaborated to create the Animal-Assisted Crisis Response National Standards (National Standards Committee for Animal-Assisted Crisis Response 2010). These standards provide concrete, specific criteria for AACR handler training, animal training, experience, evaluation and certification/registration, and standards of conduct for AACR teams. In addition to following the guidelines in the AACR National Standards, Lackey and Haberstock (2019) recommend that all AACR handlers pass four online FEMA courses—FEMA ICS-100.c, IS-700, ICS-200.b, and IS-800.c (Federal Emergency Management Agency 2008)—so that they can integrate effectively with emergency operational frameworks. To ensure appropriate training and preparation, AACR teams must seek certification or registration through a nationally recognized AACR organization. HOPE AACR (www.hopeaacr.org) and National Crisis Response Canines (https://crisisresponsecanines.org) offer handler and animal training, evaluation, and certification for handlers working exclusively with canines. The Pet Partners AACR program (https://petpartners.org/act/aacr) offers training, evaluation, and registration for handlers working with one of the nine species currently eligible for Pet Partners evaluation: dogs, horses, rabbits, cats, pot-bellied pigs, llamas/alpacas, parrots, rats, and guinea pigs. To ensure that AACR teams meet standards for appropriate training and preparation, we strongly assert that animal/handler teams must obtain certification or registration through at least one of these three organizations (HOPE AACR, National Crisis Response Canines, and Pet Partners AACR) before assisting at any crisis or disaster, even if specifically invited. If readers encounter a crisis or disaster situation in their own community that may benefit from AACR support, all three organizations are equipped to help locate and deploy appropriately qualified AACR teams.

Multicultural Considerations

Competent providers of all AAIs attend to potential cultural and diversity issues relevant to human-animal interactions and companion animal relationships (Sheade and Chandler 2014; Stewart et al. 2016). Such considerations include, but are not limited to, majority and minority cultural and ethnic groups, race, gender, socioeconomic status, levels of education, and positions of privilege and oppression. Some individuals may view certain animals as pets, others may view animals as sources from a more utilitarian perspective, while others still may have spiritual or religious perspectives (Thigpen et al. 2018). Certain species, breeds, and sizes of animals may also evoke different responses in different individuals based on culture (Greenbaum 2006), including fear, cultural or historical trauma, or disgust. Although most providers of animal-assisted therapy and animal-assisted education are able to consider these factors on a case-by-case basis *before* including a particular animal, AACR handlers are rarely able to assess cultural factors before deploying to a crisis or disaster scene (Greenbaum 2006). For this reason, it is important that AACR handlers avoid assuming that all individuals enjoy human-animal interaction, are sensitive to both verbal and nonverbal indicators of consent for an animal's proximity or approach, and develop skills in accurately assessing comfortable versus uncomfortable body language during animal interactions.

Quality and Strength of Existing Evidence

The current empirical literature specific to AACR is limited compared with literature on both AAIs and crisis response. Although many concepts relevant to general AAIs may be integrated with existing knowledge and best practices in crisis response, AACR providers have few data to support or guide their work in this highly specialized area. Future directions for AACR should include focused attention to well-designed qualitative and quantitative empirical research. Empirically based knowledge on AACR outcomes, participant and provider perspectives, and practice models could help further refine training and evaluation processes for AACR teams, tailor models to increase AACR effectiveness, and develop frameworks to facilitate integration with broad-scale emergency response systems. Another important issue for professional advocacy is lack of awareness regarding highly specialized and technical skills that must be applied in order to apply ethical and effective AAIs. Including animals in human health care is growing in popularity, but significant efforts to expand training opportunities for humans and their animal partners are needed (Stewart et al. 2022). Inadequately prepared and evaluated AACR teams have the potential to cause direct harm to vulnerable individuals and present serious concerns for animal welfare and human handler well-being. When applied with appropriate training and skills, AACR is a flexible, efficient, and valuable support strategy for empowering and encouraging short-term resilience for individuals affected by crisis. We hope to see growth in future research and professional advocacy efforts so that this already valuable and positively impactful specialization may continue to improve and refine AACR preparation, application, and best practices.

Key Clinical Points

- Animal-assisted crisis response (AACR) is a flexible and engaging specialization that aligns with many crisis response models and current neurobiological knowledge of the human stress response.

- AACR requires formal training, evaluation, and certification/registration beyond what is required for other animal-assisted activity teams.

- When working with individuals or systems affected by a crisis, psychiatrists and other mental health professionals should contact Hope Animal-Assisted Crisis Response (HOPE AACR) or Pet Partners AACR for consultation and potential mobilization of an appropriately qualified AACR team in their geographic area.

- AACR is not therapy and is not intended to help survivors heal long-term symptoms of trauma.

- AACR teams assist and support the efforts of first responders but do not directly provide first responder services.

- AACR handlers must safeguard and attend to risks associated with animal welfare, scope of practice, and their own wellness.

- More empirical research is needed to fully understand AACR's efficacy as a specialized intervention.

References

Animal Assisted Intervention International: Standards and competencies. n.d. Available at: https://aai-int.org/aai/standards-of-practice. Accessed March 13, 2022.

Briere JN, Scott C: Principles of Trauma Therapy: A Guide to Symptoms, Evaluation, and Treatment, 2nd Edition. New York, Sage, 2014

Bua F: A qualitative investigation into dogs serving on animal assisted crisis response (AACR) teams: advances in crisis counselling. Unpublished doctoral dissertation, La Trobe University, Melbourne, Australia, 2013. Available at: http://arrow.latrobe.edu.au:8080/vital/access/manager/Repository/latrobe:35600. Accessed September 1, 2021.

Caplan G: Principles of Preventive Psychiatry. New York, Basic Books, 1964

Chandler CK: Animal assisted therapy with Hurricane Katrina survivors. Based on a program presented at the ACA Annual Conference and Exhibition, Honolulu, HI, March 26–30, 2008. Available at: https://www.counseling.org/resources/library/vistas/2008-V-Online-MSWord-files/Chandler.pdf. Accessed September 1, 2021.

Chandler CK: Animal Assisted Therapy in Counseling. New York, Routledge, 2017

Federal Emergency Management Agency (FEMA): ICS Resource Center: Training Program. 2008. Available at: https://training.fema.gov/emiweb/is/icsresource/trainingmaterials. Accessed September 1, 2021.

Figley C: Compassion fatigue: toward a new understanding of the costs of caring, in Secondary Traumatic Stress: Self-Care Issues for Clinicians, Researchers, and Educators. Edited by Stamm BH. Lutherville, MD, Sidran Press, 1995, pp 3–28

France K: Crisis Intervention: A Handbook of Immediate Person-to-Person Help, 6th Edition. Springfield, IL, Charles C Thomas, 2014

Greenbaum SD: Introduction to working with Animal Assisted Crisis Response animal handler teams. Int J Emerg Ment Health 8(1):49–63, 2006 16573252

International Institute for Animal Assisted Play Therapy: AAPT Professional Certification Overview Manual. 2022. Available at: https://iiaapt.org/wp-content/uploads/2021/08/1.AAPT_.PROF_.CERTIFICATION.OVERVIEW.pdf. Accessed March 4, 2022.

Kleepsies PM: Decision Making in Behavioral Emergencies: Acquiring Skill in Evaluating and Managing High-Risk Patients. Washington, DC, American Psychological Association, 2014

Lackey R, Haberstock G: Animal-assisted crisis response: offering opportunity for human resiliency during and after traumatic incidents, in Transforming Trauma: Resilience and Healing Through Our Connection to Animals. Edited by Tedeschi P, Jenkins MA. West Lafayette, IN, Purdue University Press, 2019, pp 373–389

Lazarus RS, Folkman S: Stress, Appraisal and Coping. New York, Springer, 1984

National Standards Committee for Animal-Assisted Crisis Response: Animal-Assisted Crisis Response National Standards. March 7, 2010. Available at: http://hopeaacr.org/wp-content/uploads/2010/03/AACRNationalStandards7Mar10.pdf. Accessed March 4, 2022.

Pet Partners: Standards of Practice in Animal-Assisted Interventions. Bellevue, WA, Pet Partners, 2018

Pet Partners: Animal-Assisted Crisis Response (AACR). 2019. Available at: https://petpartners.org/act/aacr. Accessed September 1, 2021.

Sheade HE, Chandler CK: Cultural diversity considerations in animal assisted counseling. VISTAS Online, 2014. Available at: https://www.counseling.org/knowledge-center/vistas/by-year2/vistas-2014/docs/default-source/vistas/article_76. Accessed September 1, 2021.

Shiloh S, Sorek G, Terkel J: Reduction of state-anxiety by petting animals in a controlled laboratory experiment. Anxiety Stress Coping 16(4):387–395, 2003

Shubert J: Therapy dogs and stress management assistance during disasters. US Army Med Dep J Apr–Jun:74–78, 2012 22388687

Siegel DJ: Mindsight: The New Science of Personal Transformation. New York, Bantam Books, 2010

Stewart LA, Chang CY, Parker LK, Grubbs N: Animal-Assisted Therapy in Counseling Competencies. Alexandria, VA, American Counseling Association, Animal-Assisted Therapy in Mental Health Interest Network, 2016. Available at: https://www.counseling.org/docs/default-source/competencies/animal-assisted-therapy-competencies-june-2016.pdf. Accessed September 1, 2021.

Stewart LA, Hakenewerth TJ, Rabinowitz P, Fowler H: Using holistic and ethical practices with emotional support animal requests. J Creat Ment Health 17(3):410–423, 2022. Available at: https://www.tandfonline.com/doi/full/10.1080/15401383.2021.1911723. Accessed September 1, 2021.

Thigpen SE, Ellis SK, Smith RG: Special Education in Juvenile Residential Facilities: Can Animals Help? Essays in Education, Vol 14, Article 20, 2018. Available at: https://openriver.winona.edu/eie/vol14/iss1/20. Accessed September 1, 2021.

van der Kolk B: The Body Keeps the Score: Brain, Mind, and Body in the Healing of Trauma. New York, Viking Penguin, 2014

5

Companion Animals in the Treatment of At-Risk and Adjudicated Youth

Lisa D. Townsend, Ph.D., LCSW
Megan K. Mueller, Ph.D.

THIS CHAPTER FOCUSES on animal-assisted interventions (AAIs) with youth in the child welfare system and those at risk for delinquency or adjudication. Such interventions have potential as preventives as well as treatments.

Prevalence and Risk Factors

Approximately 670,000 children a year experience maltreatment in the United States. Most of these suffer from neglect; however, significant numbers of young people undergo physical, sexual, and emotional abuse (Annie E. Casey Foundation n.d.).

Factors that increase the risk for delinquency sometimes overlap with those that increase the risk for abuse and neglect, such as parent-child conflict, child hyperactivity/inattention, poverty, younger age of the child (< 4 years), child or adult mental illness, family violence, economic stressors, and community violence (Centers for Disease Control and Prevention 2021). Additional factors associated with delinquency risk are neighborhood crime, socialization with delinquent peers, and gang membership (Shader 2003). Given that juvenile justice adjudications have nearly doubled since 1960, with more than 720,000 cases processed in 2019 (Hockenberry and Puzzanchera 2021), the need for effective interventions is evident.

Clinical Outcomes and Longitudinal Time Course

Childhood abuse and neglect are associated with an array of adverse outcomes, demonstrating an exponential relationship with the number of adverse events experienced. Negative outcomes include physical disabilities, depression, PTSD, substance misuse, chronic physical illness, and suicide attempts (Felitti et al. 1998). Persistent maltreatment and an impoverished environment are linked with greater likelihood of transitioning from child welfare into the juvenile justice system, particularly for older adolescent Black males (Vidal et al. 2017). Just as there are overlapping risk factors, there is considerable overlap among youth served by the mental health, child welfare, and juvenile justice systems (Grisso 2008; Youth.gov n.d.).

Overview of Existing Evidence-Based Practices

Efforts to prevent child maltreatment consist of primary, secondary, and tertiary interventions (Casey Family Programs 2018). Primary, or universal, interventions are designed to educate parents regarding child behavior and offer supports to new families. Home visitation programs provide many of these preventive services. Secondary interventions assist families identified to be at greater risk for child maltreatment—for example, parent-child interaction therapy helps parents of children with disruptive behavior disorders adopt positive behavioral approaches to discipline (Zisser and Eyberg 2010). Tertiary treatments for youth involved with the justice system are multifaceted, surrounding the youth with a network of supports at home, at school, and in their community. The strongest evidence exists for multidimensional family therapy in the treatment of adolescent substance misuse (Filges et al. 2015). Multidimensional therapy offers home-based treatment for adjudicated youth and their parents with the aim of altering individual, social, and environmental factors that promote delinquent behavior. There is strong evidentiary support for its use in reducing rearrests, psychiatric hospitalizations, and suicide attempts (Tan and Fajardo 2017).

Companion Animals in Children's Lives

Companion animals can play an important role in the lives of children by offering companionship, acceptance, and an opportunity for nurturance and responsibility for another being (Schvaneveldt et al. 2001). The importance of animal family members has long been recognized (Carr and Rockett 2017), and emerging research suggests that they may play a healing role in the lives of foster youth. Qualitative data from youth with high rates of foster care placement disruption suggest that dogs in foster homes offer support, help build self-confidence, and lay the groundwork for establishing trust with human caregivers (Carr and Rockett 2017). Although relatively understudied as compared with AAIs and animal-assisted therapy (AAT) for at-risk youth, it is critical to acknowledge the role of companion animals for foster youth, particularly during and across housing transitions.

Animal-Assisted Interventions for Maltreated or Adjudicated Youth

Despite the existence of well-evaluated programs that serve at-risk youth, many young people go on to experience deleterious outcomes. Youth who have experienced maltreatment or involvement with the juvenile justice system frequently harbor mistrust of adults, including service providers. Involving animals in interventions to improve outcomes for these youth may form a foundation for trust and enhance their responsiveness to therapeutic services. Animals are typically perceived as nonjudgmental and emotionally safe, two key qualities that are sorely needed by maltreated or adjudicated youth. Quantitative and qualitative research repeatedly shows that children have positive psychological outcomes and enhanced learning in response to interventions involving animals (Friesen 2010). Furthermore, AAIs have a high level of acceptability as a treatment option for at-risk youth (Rabbitt et al. 2015). The following sections highlight research evaluating the efficacy and feasibility of AAIs with at-risk youth.

Equine-Facilitated Psychotherapy

Horses may play a strong therapeutic role in treating at-risk youth. Equines rely on one another for companionship, information about their environment, and safety in ways that parallel human social structures (Latella and Abrams 2019). Psychotherapy with horses requires that participants observe and respond to equine social signals—for example, if one approaches a horse with waving arms and a loud voice, the horse is likely to run away. In addition, depending on the therapeutic approach, a horse can refuse a task given its large size. Working with horses involves developing a relationship based on trust. The theoretical underpinnings of equine-facilitated psychotherapy (EFP) involve being aware of emotional and behavioral signals one is sending, processing the effect of one's behavior on the horse, and adapting one's approach to engage the horse in a mutually cooperative task (Latella and Abrams 2019).

Studies indicate that EFP is feasible with at-risk youth, even those whose problems are serious enough to warrant residential treatment (Bachi et al. 2012), and meta-analyses suggest that EFP improves social functioning among at-risk youth (Wilkie et al. 2016). Bachi et al. (2012) conducted an evaluation of weekly EFP with youth in residential treatment as a result of a court mandate or child welfare involvement. Youth participated in individual sessions over the course of 7 months, grooming and riding the horses and interacting with others at the stable. Although findings did not indicate that EFP was superior to a control condition in improving trust, self-control, self-image, or life satisfaction, the EFP group had reduced rates of readjudication compared with control youth at 1-year follow-up. Additionally, EFP or interacting with farm animals has been associated with improvements in attachment security among young people in residential foster care (Balluerka et al. 2014). One study used a 12-week individual and group therapy–based intervention to help maltreated youth uncover and reshape mistrust of others (Balluerka et al. 2014). Youth participated in two overnight stays at the farm each week with the goal of forming a trusting relationship with a farm animal of their choice. Each youth selected an animal (dog, cat, horse, sheep, goat, chicken, or pig) with which to form a relationship and learned to interact with and care for the animal for the following 12 weeks. Individual and group therapies were used to assess the youth's relationship formation strategies and reflect on their approaches to forming and maintaining those relationships. The therapist explored the youth's biases and assumptions about others and themselves, worked to reshape maladaptive cognitions about relationships, and generalized that learning to interactions off the farm. Attachment security scores increased significantly from pre- to posttherapy among youth in the AAT group, although attachment outcomes did not differ significantly from those of the control youth.

Other research has shown that EFP is comparable in effectiveness to more traditional therapeutic approaches. Roberts and Honzel (2020) evaluated group EFP as an augmentation to traditional group therapy for adolescents living in a therapeutic group home secondary to emotional and behavioral difficulties. Youth participated in traditional group therapy and group EFP, engaging in grooming, riding, and obstacle courses, and feeding the horses while taking part with therapists in trauma-focused cognitive-behavioral therapy (TF-CBT). Results comparing positive and negative affect before and after traditional and EFP groups indicated similar improvements in affect for both groups, although it should be noted that youth had higher positive affect before group EFP than before traditional group therapy. Mueller and Mc-Cullough (2017) used a quasi-experimental design to evaluate the efficacy of group EFP compared with traditional group TF-CBT. Youth with trauma histories were residents or outpatients at a behavioral health treatment facility. Most of the adolescents had juvenile justice system involvement. They received either ten 2-hour group EFP sessions over the course of 12 weeks (treatment condition) or group-based TF-CBT (control). EFP sessions consisted of grooming, leading horses over poles, completing other groundwork activities, and riding. Participants in both groups showed significant improvement on standardized measures of posttraumatic stress symptoms, although the two groups did not differ significantly.

Ethnographic work suggests possible mechanisms for emotional and behavioral improvements following EFP, including building a relationship with the horse, being free to feel "vulnerable" emotions like love and empathy, and transferring social skills learned in EFP to other areas of life (Burgon 2011). However, because these interventions often vary widely in approach and implementation, more research is needed to explore specific strategies within EFP that may be effective for at-risk youth.

Individual Psychotherapy

AAT has been used extensively in the context of psychotherapy in many populations and can help to bridge gaps in trust between abused youth and adult service providers. As noted by Fine (2019), incorporating animals into psychotherapy can help establish a positive rapport between a client and a therapist and support engagement with the therapeutic process. Parish-Plass (2008) provides case study examples of how dogs, birds, rats, and hamsters facilitate connections between youth and therapists in emergency shelter and group home facilities for youth who have been removed from their homes because of abuse or neglect. The animals may serve as alternative attachment figures, providing physical comfort and relationships in which prosocial and nurturing behaviors can be practiced.

Group Psychotherapy

CBT-based group interventions involving dogs have been used with youth involved in the child welfare and juvenile justice systems. One such program combines CBT techniques, such as positive reinforcement, communication skills, and frustration tolerance, with dog obedience, agility, and trick training. Youth engage in weekly group sessions in which the main activity is teaching skills to the dogs while the therapist emphasizes formation of adaptive social skills through positive communication between the youth and the dogs (Kelly and Cozzolino 2015). Programs like these offer nonthreatening, engaging ways for youth to learn the impact of their behavior on others and practice adaptive communication strategies that can serve them in multiple areas of their lives moving forward. Randomized controlled evaluations of therapeutic outcomes suggest that dog-training interventions are associated with significant improvements in empathy compared with empowerment-based interventions for at-risk youth (Lahav et al. 2019). Quasi-experimental evaluations of group AAT with dogs suggest the potential for significant reductions in cruelty to animals among sexually abused children (Taylor et al. 2014).

Therapy Animal Visitation Programs in Residential Juvenile Justice Settings

Few studies have been conducted to evaluate the efficacy of therapy animal visitation programs on emotional and behavioral outcomes for youth in residential detention facilities. One randomized controlled trial with adolescent girls found no significant differences between therapy animal visitation and control groups in self-reported emotional functioning or staff-reported readiness for release (Conniff et al. 2005). However, during postintervention qualitative interviews, most of the adolescents indicated that they enjoyed the program, felt less lonely after participating, and believed that all residents should have the opportunity to participate. The authors noted several limitations that could have affected their research, including documented social desirability bias in youth self-report measures and brief intervention length because of difficulties obtaining administrative approvals to conduct the study in a juvenile justice setting.

Quality and Strength of Evidence for Human-Animal Interactions in At-Risk or Adjudicated Populations

Although the body of evidence for human-animal interactions (HAIs) in other areas related to youth mental health is increasing (Hediger et al. 2021; Jones et al. 2019), the question of whether animal-assisted activities (AAAs), AAIs, or AAT for at-risk youth are efficacious remains open. The number of methodologically stringent randomized controlled trials is growing—an encouraging development—and yet many questions remain unanswered. There appears to be strong evidence for canine-assisted interventions (AAIs/AAT) for childhood trauma, according to a systematic review of evidence about AAT for youth with mental health conditions (Hoagwood et al. 2017). Variability due to animal type, intervention, and outcomes was evaluated, and the authors concluded that study designs are needed that can elucidate mechanisms by which AAIs and AAT affect youth outcomes. Specific questions include how AAT brings about physiological changes and whether animal species matters. A clear need exists for a more fine-grained understanding of which animal-assisted approaches may be most effective for at-risk and/or adjudicated youth across contexts.

Human-Animal Interaction and Positive Youth Development

Much of the literature on HAI and at-risk youth has focused on the prevention or reduction of negative behaviors and outcomes. However, human-animal relationships also provide a unique opportunity for fostering ability to thrive and resilience in youth. Theories derived from a positive youth development perspective (Lerner 2012) emphasize the importance of understanding the strengths of individuals and their contexts and aligning these strengths in ways that promote ability to thrive. Interacting with animals, either through companion animals in the home or with trained therapy animals in AAT, can provide the opportunity for youth to engage in positive social connections with both animals and people. Providing opportunities to care for an animal can be a way to foster skill-building opportunities by which youth can feel confident in their abilities. This may be especially important for youth who have experienced challenges with social interactions.

Some evidence indicates that attachment to an animal is associated with social competence and prosocial behavior in youth (Dueñas et al. 2021; Jacobson and Chang 2018; Mueller 2014). For example, interacting with animals can provide an opportunity to practice positive social interactions, both with the animals and with other people. One hypothesized mechanism underlying these improvements may be animals' unique effects on emotion regulation, often a key challenge for at-risk youth (Flynn et al. 2020). If youth can regulate their emotional responses effectively and view either a pet or a therapy animal as a social resource, these interactions serve as a scaffold for building positive relationships with others in their family and community. Structured interventions involving youth-animal interactions can also provide an opportunity to develop skills that can foster confidence and self-esteem. An exemplar of this model is Green Chimneys, a school-based, trauma-informed program that employs nature-based and animal-assisted therapies to assist youth with social, emotional, and behavioral challenges. Program goals include enhancing self-esteem and social skills, as well as helping participants achieve developmental milestones needed for adulthood (Morris et al. 2019). The Green Chimneys program includes several opportunities for youth to interact with animals, nature, and the environment, and to focus on skill-building by caring for animals while practicing positive social connections with their peers and adults.

Pet Abuse and Intimate Partner Violence

Children who come into contact with the child welfare system are frequently exposed to violent behavior between adults living in the home. Typically, this involves the physical and emotional abuse of a female parent. The World Health Organization (2021) estimates that approximately 25% of women will be exposed to violence perpetrated by a partner during their lifetime. Companion pets living in these environments are exposed to this violence and are often subjected to threats, abuse, and death at the hands of the perpetrator as a means of exerting control over women and children (Loring and Bolden-Hines 2004). Fears for their pets' safety may prompt women and children to protect the animals or comply with their abusers, making it vital to assess for violence against pets and threats of harm to pets as an important component of safety planning for families involved with the child welfare system (Ascione 2000). One option for promoting animal welfare and protecting abused youth may be collaborative linkages between child welfare and animal abuse organizations. A study that evaluated cross-reporting of suspected child and animal abuse or neglect reported overlap between instances of both types of abuse (children's services workers reported animal welfare concerns in 20% of homes visited, and humane society workers reported child welfare concerns in 10% of homes visited; Zilney and Zilney 2005).

Clinical and Animal Welfare Considerations

Employing evidence-based practices for maintaining animal safety, welfare, and well-being is critical in conducting interventions involving animals in an ethical manner (Ng et al. 2019). Screening potential program participants is an important step in protecting the welfare of animal participants and maximizing potential intervention benefits, given that youth who have experienced abuse may be at higher risk for harming animals. When comparing rates of animal abuse by children who experienced no abuse (normative sample) with those in a child psychiatric sample and those among children who experienced sexual abuse, Ascione et al. (2003) found that rates of parent-reported animal abuse were 17.9% among sexually abused children, 15.6% among a child psychiatric sample, and 3.1% in the normative sample. Gender differences in rates of animal abuse indicated higher rates of animal abuse among sexually abused boys (25%) compared with girls (6.1%). In both the sexually abused and the psychiatric samples, rates of animal abuse were higher when physical abuse was also present. Similar findings have been documented in longitudinal studies of children who have experienced harsh parenting strategies (Becker et al. 2004).

For youth who may be at risk for animal abuse or who have behavioral or emotion regulation challenges, taking a proactive approach to ensuring animal and human safety in AAIs is critical. Green Chimneys' approach to safety provides an example of strategies for protecting child and animal welfare during therapeutic interactions (Morris et al. 2019). Collaboration between clinicians and animal handlers/professionals is a key element of success, as is a shared understanding of human and animal behaviors that could lead to welfare or safety concerns. An individual approach to understanding each child's history with animals and potential risk for unsafe behaviors can be used to develop an appropriate plan for engaging with animals safely. Before youth interact with animals, clinicians and staff should be trained to assess whether any dysregulation or potentially risky behaviors are occurring and, if needed, provide either a nonanimal alternative or deescalation support prior to animal engagement. The Green Chimneys model also includes an Animal Safety Committee, which can assess risk prior to HAI and create a safe remediation plan for reintegration if necessary (Morris et al. 2019). This individualized approach allows for protecting the safety of the animals and people involved, as well as maximizing the potential for success of the intervention by creating contexts that are appropriate for individual children based on their challenges, strengths, and therapeutic needs.

Areas for Future Research

Evidence suggests that AAIs involving horses and dogs are feasible and received well by at-risk or adjudicated youth and are linked with some positive outcomes. However, more randomized controlled trials are needed to establish a stronger foundation for AAAs, AAIs, and AAT in this population and to isolate mechanisms of effect. Furthermore, little work has been done to establish a role for these interventions in promoting long-term positive outcomes.

In addition, relatively little research has been done on companion animal ownership for at-risk youth. Although pets have the potential to provide emotional support and foster resilience in the context of adversity (Applebaum et al. 2021), the specific role of companion animals for youth who have challenging family situations has not been well studied. Some initial research with adult populations has shown that attachment to pets plays a key role during family conflict (Applebaum and Zsembik 2020), but further work with youth samples is needed to establish the precise protective role, if any, of pets in different family circumstances.

When working with at-risk youth and animals, it is important for practitioners to take a person-centered approach to addressing potential challenges that come up when working with animals. For example, consider the following:

Case Example

Evan, a 10-year-old boy, had several diagnoses (including autism spectrum disorder) and challenges with behavioral and emotion regulation. Evan was participating in an AAT intervention at school, where his speech-language pathologist (SLP) was partnering with a therapy animal handler and her experienced therapy dog partner, Greta. Before beginning AAT, the treatment team had conducted a risk assessment and created a safety plan, which included the presence of Evan's paraprofessional aide in addition to the SLP and therapy dog handler, to supervise all aspects of the interaction. Generally, Evan responded well to interacting with the therapy dog, and the SLP found that when the therapy dog was present, Evan was more engaged in his speech exercises. However, during one of the sessions, Evan became frustrated and attempted to hit Greta.

The therapy dog handler was engaging in best practices, which included staying in close proximity to her dog, and therefore she was able to remove Greta from the situation immediately without any harm to the dog. The clinician and paraprofessional were also engaging in the predetermined safety plan guidelines by closely monitoring Evan's behavior and were able to safely move him to another location and de-escalate. Following this incident, the collaborative team met to reevaluate their safety plan and assess if they could safely reengage with the therapy dog. The team determined that Evan benefited from engaging with Greta but that a staged approach to reintroducing therapy dog interaction was necessary to maintain a safe environment for both Evan and Greta and that additional safeguards would be put into place. They developed an individual plan for Evan, which included the following three steps:

1. **Allow for a temporary period when Evan can practice interacting appropriately with a dog using a stuffed dog.** The focus was on positive engagement, emotion regulation, and learning verbal and hand commands that Evan could give from a distance (e.g., sit, down).

2. **Reintroduce interactions with Greta, with engagement from a distance.** The handler was able to keep Greta out of reach, while Evan practiced safely engaging with verbal and hand commands with Greta.

3. **Reintroduce physical interaction as Evan is able to demonstrate regulated behavior around Greta.** Interactions were highly supervised, and the SLP and accompanying paraprofessional aide monitored Evan's behavioral and emotion regulation carefully and in close proximity. Evan's behavior and emotional state were assessed prior to the start of each session to ensure that interaction with Greta would be appropriate on that day. If Evan began to become dysregulated, Greta was calmly moved to a safe location. The therapy dog handler continuously monitored Greta's behavior and would remove her if any stress signals occurred.

By using this staged approach, the practitioner and handler team were able to safely reintroduce therapy dog interactions with Evan. The important components of the plan were 1) taking an individualized approach to Evan's behavioral needs with professionals who knew his challenges and strengths; 2) working collaboratively with the animal handler to create a plan that would be safe for the therapy dog and allowed continuous monitoring of dog safety and stress; 3) taking a gradual approach to build the skills necessary for safe interactions, including beginning with nonphysical interactions; and 4) ensuring communication and clarity among the treatment team regarding when interactions should be stopped for safety.

This case example underscores the need for thorough risk assessment and planning when AAIs are being conducted in order to safeguard the welfare of the animals and people involved. Assessment tools to guide safety planning, such as the Lincoln Education Assistance with Dogs (LEAD) Risk Assessment Tool (Brelsford et al. 2020), are available. The LEAD instrument can inform safety planning discussions with staff, including reviewing sources of risk and assigning designees responsible for mitigating them. Key considerations include characterizing the likelihood of aggression prior to initiating an AAI with at-risk or adjudicated youth, ensuring a high level of supervision during activities and interventions, and implementing multiple layers of protection within the program's framework. One example of multilayered protections is in the Diamond Model of AAI (MacNamara et al. 2019), which includes the dog, handler, clinician, and patient. The handler assumes primary responsibility for the dog's welfare during the session and collaborates with the therapist to ensure that therapeutic activities do not stress or harm the animal. The clinician assumes primary responsibility for the patient. Safety plans should be continuously reassessed, particularly if any behavior occurs that elevates risk for human or animal participants.

Additional levels of protection can be conferred by documenting a patient's history of aggression toward people and animals as well as carrying out a presession risk assessment that characterizes a youth's current level of emotional or behavioral dysregulation and recent stressors that could function as antecedents for aggressive behavior. If one or more of these indicators are present prior to an intervention, session activities can be altered accordingly to minimize risk to animals or people. Therapy animal handlers should always be encouraged to remove their animals if they feel that the situation is not comfortable for their animals.

Key Clinical Points

- Animal-assisted interventions (AAIs) are feasible and associated with positive outcomes among some at-risk youth.

- More rigorous scientific research is needed to evaluate the efficacy of AAIs and animal-assisted therapies for at-risk youth and to tailor interventions to address their unique needs.

- Thorough risk assessment and multilayered safety plans that focus on animal and human safety are critical.

Screening for aggression toward animals and developing an appropriate safety plan for individual youth are key components of providing for the safety of animals involved in AAIs.

- Cross-reporting between animal and child welfare agencies could facilitate identification of undetected abuse or neglect of children and animals.

- Pets may play an important role in supporting resilience within the family context for at-risk youth, but further research is needed.

References

Annie E. Casey Foundation: Child protection. n.d. Available at: www.aecf.org/topics/child-protection. Accessed December 3, 2021.

Applebaum JW, Zsembik BA: Pet attachment in the context of family conflict. Anthrozoos 33(3):361–370, 2020

Applebaum JW, MacLean EL, McDonald SE: Love, fear, and the human-animal bond: on adversity and multispecies relationships. Compr Psychoneuroendocrinol 7:100071, 2021 34485952

Ascione FR: Safe havens for pets: guidelines for programs sheltering pets for women who are battered. 2000. Available at: https://lucysproject.com.au/wp-content/uploads/Safe-Havens-for-Pets-Frank-R-Ascione.pdf. Accessed March 19, 2022.

Ascione FR, Friedrich WN, Heath J, Hayashi K: Cruelty to animals in normative, sexually abused, and outpatient psychiatric samples of 6- to 12-year-old children: relations to maltreatment and exposure to domestic violence. Anthrozoos 16(3):194–212, 2003

Bachi K, Terkel J, Teichman M: Equine-facilitated psychotherapy for at-risk adolescents: the influence on self-image, self-control and trust. Clin Child Psychol Psychiatry 17(2):298–312, 2012 21757481

Balluerka N, Muela A, Amiano N, Caldentey MA: Influence of animal-assisted therapy (AAT) on the attachment representations of youth in residential care. Child Youth Serv Rev 42:103–109, 2014

Becker KD, Stuewig J, Herrera VM, McCloskey LA: A study of firesetting and animal cruelty in children: family influences and adolescent outcomes. J Am Acad Child Adolesc Psychiatry 43(7):905–912, 2004 15213592

Brelsford VL, Dimolareva M, Gee NR, Meints K: Best practice standards in animal-assisted interventions: how the *LEAD* Risk Assessment Tool can help. Animals (Basel) 10(6):974, 2020 32503309

Burgon HL: "Queen of the world": experiences of "at-risk" young people participating in equine-assisted learning/therapy. J Soc Work Pract 25(2):165–183, 2011

Carr S, Rockett B: Fostering secure attachment: experiences of animal companions in the foster home. Attach Hum Dev 19(3):259–277, 2017 28277096

Casey Family Programs: What are some examples of evidence-informed practices to keep children safe and promote permanency? February 6, 2018. Available at: https://www.casey.org/what-are-some-examples-of-evidence-informed-practices-to-keep-children-safe-and-promote-permanency. Accessed March 19, 2022.

Centers for Disease Control and Prevention: Violence prevention: risk and protective factors. 2021. Available at: https://www.cdc.gov/violenceprevention/childabuseandneglect/riskprotectivefactors.html. Accessed March 19, 2022.

Conniff KM, Scarlett JM, Goodman S, Appel LD: Effects of a pet visitation program on the behavior and emotional state of adjudicated female adolescents. Anthrozoos 18(4):379–395, 2005

Dueñas J-M, Gonzàlez L, Forcada R, et al: The relationship between living with dogs and social and emotional development in childhood. Anthrozoos 34(1):33–46, 2021

Felitti VJ, Anda RF, Nordenberg D, et al: Relationship of childhood abuse and household dysfunction to many of the leading causes of death in adults: the Adverse Childhood Experiences (ACE) Study. Am J Prev Med 14(4):245–258, 1998 9635069

Filges T, Rasmussen PS, Andersen D, Jørgensen A-MK: Multidimensional Family Therapy (MDFT) for young people in treatment for non-opioid drug abuse: a systematic review. Campbell Syst Rev 11(1):1–124, 2015

Fine AH: Incorporating animal-assisted interventions into psychotherapy guidelines and suggestions for therapists, in Handbook on Animal-Assisted Therapy: Foundations and Guidelines for Animal-Assisted Interventions, 5th Edition. Edited by Fine AH. London, Elsevier Academic Press, 2019, pp 207–224

Flynn E, Mueller MK, Luft D, et al: Human-animal-environment interactions and self-regulation in youth with psychosocial challenges: initial assessment of the Green Chimneys model. Hum Anim Interact Bull 8(2):55–67, 2020

Friesen L: Exploring animal-assisted programs with children in school and therapeutic contexts. Early Child Educ J 37(4):261–267, 2010

Grisso T: Adolescent offenders with mental disorders. Future Child 18(2):143–164, 2008 21338001

Hediger K, Wagner J, Künzi P, et al: Effectiveness of animal-assisted interventions for children and adults with post-traumatic stress disorder symptoms: a systematic review and meta-analysis. Eur J Psychotraumatol 12(1):1879713, 2021 34377357

Hoagwood KE, Acri M, Morrissey M, Peth-Pierce R: Animal-assisted therapies for youth with or at risk for mental health problems: a systematic review. Appl Dev Sci 21(1):1–13, 2017 28798541

Hockenberry S, Puzzanchera C: Juvenile Court Statistics 2019. Pittsburgh, PA, National Center for Juvenile Justice, 2021. Available at: https://www.ojjdp.gov/ojstatbb/njcda/pdf/jcs2019.pdf. Accessed March 18, 2022.

Jacobson KC, Chang L: Associations between pet ownership and attitudes toward pets with youth socioemotional outcomes. Front Psychol 9:2304, 2018 30534102

Jones MG, Rice SM, Cotton SM: Incorporating animal-assisted therapy in mental health treatments for adolescents: a systematic review of canine assisted psychotherapy. PLoS One 14(1):e0210761, 2019 30653587

Kelly MA, Cozzolino CA: Helping at-risk youth overcome trauma and substance abuse through animal-assisted therapy. Contemporary Justice Review 18(4):421–434, 2015

Lahav S, Sarid O, Kantor H: Effects of a dog-training intervention on at-risk youth. Anthrozoos 32(4):533–540, 2019

Latella D, Abrams B: The role of the equine in animal-assisted interactions, in Handbook on Animal-Assisted Therapy: Foundations and Guidelines for Animal-Assisted Interventions, 5th Edition. Edited by Fine AH. London, Elsevier Academic Press, 2019, pp 133–162

Lerner RM: Developmental science: past, present, and future. Int J Dev Sci 6(1–2):29–36, 2012

Loring MT, Bolden-Hines TA: Pet abuse by batterers as a means of coercing battered women into committing illegal behavior. Journal of Emotional Abuse 4(1):27–37, 2004

MacNamara M, Moga J, Pachel C: What's love got to do with it? Selecting animals for animal-assisted mental health interventions, in Handbook on Animal-Assisted Therapy: Foundations and Guidelines for Animal-Assisted Interventions, 5th Edition. Edited by Fine AH. London, Elsevier Academic Press, 2019, pp 101–113

Morris KN, Flynn E, Jenkins MA, et al: Documentation of Nature-Based Programs at Green Chimneys. Denver, CO, University of Denver, Institute for Human-Animal Connection, 2019. Available at: https://www.greenchimneys.org/wp-content/uploads/2020/01/IHAC_Green-Chimneys-Program-Documentation_-2019.pdf. Accessed March 19, 2022.

Mueller MK: Is human-animal interaction (HAI) linked to positive youth development? Initial answers. Appl Dev Sci 18(1):5–16, 2014

Mueller MK, McCullough L: Effects of equine-facilitated psychotherapy on post-traumatic stress symptoms in youth. J Child Fam Stud 26(4):1164–1172, 2017

Ng ZY, Albright JD, Fine AH, Peralta JM: Our ethical and moral responsibility, in Handbook on Animal-Assisted Therapy: Foundations and Guidelines for Animal-Assisted Interventions, 5th Edition. Edited by Fine AH. London, Elsevier Academic Press, 2019, pp 175–198

Parish-Plass N: Animal-assisted therapy with children suffering from insecure attachment due to abuse and neglect: a method to lower the risk of intergenerational transmission of abuse? Clin Child Psychol Psychiatry 13(1):7–30, 2008 18411863

Rabbitt SM, Kazdin AE, Hong JE: Acceptability of animal-assisted therapy: attitudes toward AAT, psychotherapy, and medication for the treatment of child disruptive behavioral problems. Anthrozoos 27(3):335–350, 2015

Roberts H, Honzel N: The effectiveness of equine-facilitated psychotherapy in adolescents with serious emotional disturbances. Anthrozoos 33(1):133–144, 2020

Schvaneveldt PL, Young MH, Schvaneveldt JD, Kivett VR: Interaction of people and pets in the family setting: a life course perspective. Journal of Teaching in Marriage and Family 1(2):34–51, 2001

Shader M: Risk factors for delinquency: an overview. Washington, DC, Office of Juvenile Justice and Delinquency Prevention, 2003. Available at: https://www.ojp.gov/ncjrs/virtual-library/abstracts/risk-factors-delinquency-overview. Accessed March 19, 2022.

Tan JX, Fajardo MLR: Efficacy of multisystemic therapy in youths aged 10-17 with severe antisocial behaviour and emotional disorders: systematic review. London J Prim Care (Abingdon) 9(6):95–103, 2017 29181092

Taylor N, Fraser H, Signal T, Prentice K: Social work, animal-assisted therapies and ethical considerations: a programme example from Central Queensland, Australia. Br J Soc Work 46(1):135–152, 2014

Vidal S, Prince D, Connell CM, et al: Maltreatment, family environment, and social risk factors: determinants of the child welfare to juvenile justice transition among maltreated children and adolescents. Child Abuse Negl 63:7–18, 2017 27886518

Wilkie KD, Germain S, Theule J: Evaluating the efficacy of equine therapy among at-risk youth: a meta-analysis. Anthrozoos 29(3):377–393, 2016

World Health Organization: Violence against women. March 9, 2021. Available at: https://www.who.int/news-room/fact-sheets/detail/violence-against-women. Accessed March 19, 2022.

Youth.gov: Connections with youth in the child welfare system. n.d. Available at: https://youth.gov/youth-topics/juvenile-justice/connections-youth-child-welfare-system. Accessed March 19, 2022.

Zilney LA, Zilney M: Reunification of child and animal welfare agencies: cross-reporting of abuse in Wellington County, Ontario. Child Welfare 84(1):47–66, 2005 15717773

Zisser A, Eyberg SM: Parent-child interaction therapy and the treatment of disruptive behavior disorders, in Evidence-Based Psychotherapies for Children and Adolescents, 2nd Edition. New York, Guilford, 2010, pp 179–193

6

Companion Animals in the Treatment of ADHD

Sabrina E. B. Schuck, Ph.D.
Ann Childress, M.D.

MEDIA ATTENTION and reports have described how dogs are purported to provide a wide range of support and services for children (e.g., visiting preschools and children's hospitals, community library reading programs), driving public demand for these kinds of opportunities. As this demand has increased rapidly, so too has the need for standardized guidelines and more rigorous empirical evidence for these practices. In the last decade, research has also increased on the study of human-animal interaction (HAI), and particularly on the effect of animal-assisted interventions (AAIs). Still, this work is nascent, and information about these practices is not widely available to health care professionals and consumers.

Perhaps as a result of this mainstream attention, parents of children with neurodevelopmental disorders are increasingly acquiring pets for their children and expecting a therapeutic benefit from pet ownership (Carlisle 2015; Crossman and Kazdin 2016). Despite the popularity of these practices, little is still known about the efficacy of AAIs and pet ownership for young children with ADHD and related behavior problems. In this chapter, we provide an overview of the state of the science on AAIs and pet ownership, as well as suggestions for providers and family members based on our current understanding of that science.

Prevalence of ADHD

ADHD is the most prevalent childhood psychiatric condition, with a worldwide prevalence estimate between 5.0% and 7.2% (Faraone et al. 2003), affecting nearly 9.4% of children in the United States (Danielson et al. 2017). The annual cost of ADHD is estimated at $266 billion, much of which is lost productivity and income for adults with ADHD and parents of children who have ADHD (Doshi et al. 2012). Despite decades of research aimed at optimizing outcomes for children with ADHD, the condition remains a significant public health problem adversely affecting individuals, families, and schools (Robb et al. 2011).

Clinical Presentation and Longitudinal Time Course

A childhood diagnosis of ADHD has long been associated with the later development of comorbid mental disorders and poor health outcomes related to problems with self-regulation, such as early substance use, risky sexual behavior, and dangerous driving (Flory et al. 2006; Molina and Pelham 2003; Thompson et al. 2007). Symptoms of inattention and hyperactive/impulsive behaviors present in individuals with ADHD early in childhood and often persist across the life span (Caye et al. 2016). A longitudinal examination over more than a decade found that childhood ADHD resulted in atypically early substance use and was especially associated with increased risk for habitual (daily) smoking (Howard et al. 2020). Furthermore, persisting problems with self-regulation are associated with greater risk for school failure or attrition (Trampush et al. 2009).

Overview of Existing Evidence-Based Interventions

Pharmacological management of ADHD symptoms is recommended as a first-line treatment in patients age 6 years or older (Wolraich et al. 2019). Both stimulants (methylphenidate and amphetamine) and non-stimulants (atomoxetine, clonidine extended release [ER], guanfacine ER, and viloxazine ER) are FDA approved to treat ADHD (Wolraich et al. 2019). Stimulants are the most effective of the pharmacological agents, with 68%–97% of patients responding to either methylphenidate or amphetamine (Hodgkins et al. 2012). Although both stimulant and nonstimulant medications have been found to reduce symptoms of ADHD, effect sizes for change are greater for stimulants (Joseph et al. 2017). Approximately 30 different formulations of amphetamine and methylphenidate are available to treat ADHD, and multiple ER formulations have been developed in the last two decades that differ in technology used to control the release and delivery of the drug (Steingard et al. 2019). Stimulants are available as capsules, chewable and oral disintegrating tablets, liquid suspensions, and a dermal patch. These formulations have varied pharmacokinetic profiles that control onset and duration of efficacy (Childress et al. 2019).

Catalá-López et al. (2017) published a systematic review of treatments for ADHD that employed a network meta-analysis of randomized controlled trials. This review found that at the class level, behavioral therapy in combination with stimulants was superior to medications alone (stimulants or nonstimulants). Treatment with stimulants alone was found to be superior to nonstimulants alone, behavioral therapy alone, and cognitive training alone. The best profile for treatment acceptability was the combination of behavioral therapy and stimulants.

Contraindications for Pharmacological Intervention

Pharmacological treatment to decrease symptoms is the mainstay of traditional intervention for ADHD, but adherence to these treatments is poor and failures are common (Caye et al. 2019; Schneider and Enenbach 2014). Furthermore, product labels list numerous warnings and precautions. Despite the varied delivery systems available, a considerable number of patients may have difficulty with tolerability of stimulants and nonstimulants (Cortese et al. 2018). Stimulants, atomoxetine, and viloxazine may increase blood pressure (Takeda Pharmaceuticals 2021). Furthermore, concomitant use of drugs that decrease blood pressure and heart rate should be avoided when the patient is taking guanfacine ER or clonidine ER (Concordia Pharmaceuticals 2020; Shire U.S. 2019). Both atomoxetine and viloxazine ER have warnings for suicidal thoughts and behaviors, which are not common but occurred more often with the drugs than with placebo in controlled trials.

There is also evidence of limited effectiveness of medicines as children age (MTA Cooperative Group 2004). More recently, there are concerns about long-term adverse effects of stimulant treatment, including effects on growth (Carucci et al. 2021) and body mass (Baweja et al. 2021). Of interest, when children do benefit from treatment with medications, research indicates that those who also had behavioral interventions (i.e., behavioral parent training and brief teacher consultation) prior to medication treatment fared better than those who received medication first (Pelham et al. 2016).

Although treatment effect sizes of nonpharmacological interventions for reducing symptoms are not as large as those for treatment with stimulants, well-established evidence supports psychosocial interventions for children with ADHD, including behavioral parent education, social skills training, and school support services (Fabiano et al. 2015). Despite this evidence, significantly more barriers exist to accessing psychosocial interventions when compared with medication treatment (Danielson et al. 2017). Although psychosocial interventions have been found to provide short-term treatment gains, promoting generalizability of those gains is less well understood (Green and Langberg 2022). Furthermore, these treatment gains are generally found to diminish over time without "boosters"; thus, continued treatment combined with medication management is thought to best support benefits over time (Antshel 2015).

Animal-Assisted Interventions as an Integrative Strategy for ADHD

Yerkes and Dodson's (1908) early theories of learning argue that cognitive or mental arousal must be optimal for learning to take place, and the relationship between emotion, motivation, and attention and learning has long been established (Cahill et al. 1994). Parents and teachers anecdotally report that animals motivate children to perform tasks otherwise avoided, acting as a catalyst for improving engagement and sustained attention in difficult and/or nonpreferred tasks (Gee et al. 2015). HAI literature describes beneficial cognitive and physiological findings across different populations of children with and without neurodevelopmental disorders (Becker et al. 2017; O'Haire et al. 2013). In a study of neurotypically developing children, when dogs were integrated into classrooms, children had fewer behavioral difficulties and stayed on task longer (Kotrschal and Ortbauer 2003).

Of particular interest for the field of ADHD intervention, some skills of executive functioning in typically developing preschool children, particularly working memory, were found to be improved when a therapy dog was in the room (Gee et al. 2010). More recently, therapeutic horseback riding was found to improve skills of executive functioning and self-esteem among children with ADHD (Aviv et al. 2021). These findings are particularly compelling for informing specific ways that different species can be integrated into clinical practice with evidence-based therapies and helping determine which deficits AAIs may most effectively target. Our current understanding of the executive functioning deficits that are a hallmark of ADHD, considered together with recent findings on the effects of animals in classroom and therapeutic settings, supports the concept that AAI may bring about positive change in skills of executive functioning for children with ADHD. Although the mechanisms of action are not well understood, interaction with a dog may act on physiological systems affecting executive functioning in ways similar to the strategies implemented in behavioral token economy systems—motivating attention, eliciting emotion, and thereby optimizing cognitive arousal and stamina to promote learning and generalization.

For children with ADHD, for whom attention is difficult to arouse and sustain, interaction with a dog may not only help capture attention (i.e., the metaphorical "hook" for pulling a child into a learning or therapeutic experience) but also sustain attention, thereby facilitating meaningful learning from more traditional therapies. Theoretically, in keeping with McGaugh's (2006) descriptions of arousal and memory, the animal accompanying otherwise less memorable interventions elicits the "arousal" that "makes mild moments memorable."

Quality and Strength of Existing Evidence for Animal-Assisted Interventions as Treatment

Considering the limitations of evidence-based practices for treating ADHD, it is not surprising that many parents continue to seek alternative and complementary interventions for ADHD. Of interest, parents have reported finding AAIs to be more acceptable than medication for children with disruptive behavior problems (Rabbitt et al. 2014). A recent systematic review focusing on the inclusion of an AAI with dogs in psychotherapy across settings reported emerging evidence in the field suggesting that this practice is acceptable, tolerable, and feasible and improves the efficacy of mental health treatments in self-selected adolescent populations (Jones et al. 2019).

Historically, systematic research examining these practices and publication of related scholarly works have been sparse. The past decade, however, has seen a significant increase in both the quality and the quantity of research, particularly on AAIs with children who have special needs. Burgeoning evidence supports the efficacy of AAIs for reducing stress and improving social skills across special populations, especially in children with autism spectrum disorders (for a discussion of this work, see Chapter 7, "Companion Animals in the Treatment of Autism Spectrum Disorder"). By comparison, however, relatively little research allows for systematic review of these practices for children who have ADHD. In a recent search in Google Scholar, the terms *ADHD* and *animal-assisted therapy* (AAT) retrieved 940 results for works since 2017, whereas a similar search for *autism* retrieved 2,590 results in the same time frame. Furthermore, the vast majority of scholarly publications on animal-assisted practices and children specifically with ADHD are reviews (e.g., Selamat et al. 2018), commentary, small case studies, or student papers (e.g., Valley-Damkoehler 2019). Isolated case studies (Juríčková et al. 2020) and small intervention studies (Gilboa and Helmer 2020) describe promising results but lack randomization and adequate control conditions to inform clinical practice.

A small pre-post design study examined a self-management occupational therapy AAI with horses for children with ADHD ($N=25$, ages 6–14 years) (Gilboa and Helmer 2020). This intervention targeted executive functioning skills and found significant improvements across several domains. Findings of this study are limited by the small sample size and the lack of a control condition but are of interest in that improvements occurred, specifically in skills of working memory ($t=2.476$; $P=0.021$). In a systematic review of AAT for a broad group of youth with or at risk for mental health problems, Hoagwood et al. (2017) reviewed all experimental AAT studies published between 2000 and 2015. This work compared studies by animal type, intervention, and outcomes. Notably, of the 24 studies identified, only 11 used randomized controlled trials, with most of those addressing equine therapies for autism spectrum disorder.

In another systematic review that focused on both qualitative and quantitative studies specifically incorporating dogs into mental health treatments and psychosocial outcomes for adolescents (ages 10–19 years) with a variety of diagnostic presentations, researchers found only seven studies meeting inclusion criteria (Jones et al. 2019). Overall, psychotherapy assisted by dogs was found to have a positive effect on reducing symptomatology, conferring additional benefits over standard treatments for internalizing disorders and PTSD and equivalent effects for anxiety, anger, and externalizing disorders. Notably, the AAI with dogs was associated with effects on secondary factors including increased engagement and socialization behaviors and reductions in disruptive be-haviors within treatment sessions.

In summary, numerous works point to positive effects of AAIs for children with mental health conditions. However, there are few well-controlled and adequately powered clinical trials evaluating objective outcomes as well as the more subjective reports of caregivers and teach-ers. Additionally, there is little information about what kinds of AAIs are most effective and for whom. These gaps in our understanding of AAIs indicate that considerable work remains to be done before clinicians can recommend these practices as a part of an integrative therapy for indi-viduals with ADHD.

Randomized Controlled Trial of ADHD and Animal-Assisted Intervention: Safety, Acceptability, Feasibility, and Efficacy

The first randomized controlled trial examining the safety and efficacy of an AAI for children with ADHD—the Positive Assertive Cooperative Kids (PACK) study—was funded by the Eunice Kennedy Shriver National In-stitute of Child Health and Human Development in 2010 (R01HD66593). A total of 88 medication-naive children with ADHD, ages 7–9 years, and their parents participated. With a rigorously controlled study design and standardized treatment protocol (see Schuck et al. 2018a for more detail), both AAI and nonpharmacological treatment as usual were found acceptable and feasibly deployed (98% and 91% respective reten-tion rates at follow-up). Notably, both interventions were found to be safe, with no adverse events reported for children, staff, handlers, or dogs over the 4-year study period. Results of that study indicated that outcomes were modestly enhanced by the assistance of therapy dogs (AAI) when compared with the treatment-as-usual intervention (Schuck et al. 2018a, 2018b), with both groups reporting significant reductions in parent ratings of ADHD symptom severity over time ($P < 0.0001$). Of note, significant group differences emerged early at 2 weeks into the in-tervention, holding through week 8, such that ratings were significantly lower in the AAI group when compared with the treatment-as-usual group ($P < 0.05$), with a moderate effect size ($d = 0.54$). Symptom severity remained lower in the AAI group at week 10 ($P < 0.05$), with a small to moderate effect size ($d = 0.38$), and this trend held at week 12 (at 54 hours); however, the difference was no longer significant ($P = 0.06$).

Findings from the PACK study are promising and suggest that AAIs may be a viable integrative treatment strategy for enhancing and generalizing treatment gains from psychosocial interventions in school-based settings. Practically speaking, after-school programs or school visitation programs that incorporate trained therapy dogs into behavioral therapies emphasizing the development of social skills can be feasibly and safely provided by behavioral health professionals in conjunction with volunteer therapy animal organizations. Until this study, there had not been any fully powered and randomized controlled trials providing evidence for AAIs for ADHD. These findings of the PACK study are particularly compelling because treatment options for ADHD, especially for symptoms of inattention, have not changed significantly for decades.

Animal-Assisted Intervention Practices for Children With ADHD

Children with ADHD often present with relatively impaired skills of executive functioning (e.g., self-regulation) and poor self-awareness when compared with their typically developing peers. Common treatment aims include improving executive functioning skills. A first step to implementing established evidence-based psychosocial interventions for children with ADHD is to use a cognitive-behavioral approach for improving self-awareness through feedback with the goals of improving attention, inhibition, and working memory.

The intervention described in the PACK study used three main AAI practices specifically designed to complement cognitive-behavioral strategies and psychosocial therapies previously found effective for ADHD (Schuck et al. 2015). Key elements of these practices included a structured social skills training curriculum preceded by an unstructured "bonding" time, complemented with structured dog-themed activities typically used in schools. Children then participated in a lesson from a manualized dog-training program developed by the investigators (Schuck et al. 2013) incorporating lessons inspired by the American Humane Society's *Kids Interacting With Dogs Safely* workbook (Deming et al. 2009) with the psychosocial skills training strategies implemented in the Multimodal Treatment Study of ADHD (Wells et al. 2000). These practices were assisted by trained therapy dog/handler dyads selected for this work through a multilevel screening process.

Animal-child "bonding" opportunities were provided when the children arrived at the sessions and were aimed at building the child-animal relationship during unstructured, noncontingent "stations" at various places in the facility (e.g., yard, rug) where children could stop by and interact in a dog-preferred activity (e.g., agility, obedience, grooming). Children moved among activities prior to starting structured psycho-social skills training sessions.

These sessions also included an animal-assisted education lesson or activity aimed at improving skills of reading and writing. Inattention is generally considered to be the most impairing symptom of ADHD that persists across the life span (Franke et al. 2018). Therefore, common treatment goals for practitioners include *engaging and sustaining attention*, with the aim of increasing task completion and building adaptive skills necessary for school or occupational success. A related treatment goal is to *increase the amount of time children spend on nonpreferred tasks*, and particularly tasks that require *sustained mental effort*, which are often avoided in school (e.g., reading and writing). To this end, the PACK study treatment protocol used an animal-assisted education lesson or activity strategies targeting these goals coupled with the simple presence of a therapy dog and handler during these practices. Specifically, dog-themed reading and writing exercises were implemented during therapy sessions in which children sat on the classroom floor in small groups, each next to one dyad, to listen to a story read aloud by a behavioral therapist. On subsequent occasions, children were asked to read aloud from an age- and reading-level-matched passage in small groups containing a few children and a dog. Later, children were asked to write in a journal about something they had learned about the dogs during the intervention. Finally, children were instructed to write a letter to one of the therapy dogs when the dogs were not present.

PACK sessions included a structured and manualized dog-training lesson in which the children would practice teaching basic commands to experienced therapy dogs; this lesson was aimed specifically at helping to influence planning, to improve self-regulation, and to implement goal-directed activity. Although hyperactivity and impulsivity decrease over time for many individuals with ADHD, many report a continued sense of restlessness and difficulty waiting in adulthood. Those with more severe symptoms of hyperactivity/impulsivity in childhood are at greater risk for the development of comorbid disorders that result in substantial impairment, including substance abuse disorders and mood disorders. Central to these areas of impairment are poor self-regulation and impaired social relationships. Thus, common treatment goals include *increased compliance with rules and directions* and *increased frustration tolerance*. The PACK study developed structured ways in which the use of therapy dogs could enhance more traditional skills training by incorporating dog "training" to target treatment goals. In each lesson, children were first taught a specific social skill through discussion and role-play (e.g., assertion, accepting) and were then instructed to teach simple commands to the therapy dogs—or "How to Be a Good Teacher" of dogs. These dog-training lessons included a review of animal/dog safety, an emphasis on humane treatment of animals, and instruction on how to consider the dog's perspective. Lessons focused on basic commands that therapy dogs are experienced in performing for their handlers (e.g., sit, stay, come) but that they may be less likely to perform for children. Practices emphasized planning, self-regulation, and persistence in the face of frustration while encouraging children to identify thoughts and feelings during exercises (Schuck et al. 2013). Children were later counseled about how they might plan to manage challenges in the next session.

Settings for Animal-Assisted Interventions, Therapies, and Activities

Although recent research suggests that involving animals in therapeutic settings, particularly dogs and horses, is beneficial for children with ADHD, significantly less is known about the role of pets in the home for these children. Similarly, little is known about the role of individual differences in pet preferences, cultural attitudes and beliefs about pets, and self-referral biases in determining the effectiveness of pet ownership and long-term outcomes for these children. Furthermore, there is scant research comparing the effectiveness of different animal species with this group of children (Brelsford et al. 2017) and even less research examining the effect of the relative temperament of different animals in interventions (Bray et al. 2020).

No evidence supports bringing a dog into a home under the premise that the animal will provide therapeutic benefit to a child with ADHD. On the contrary, providing necessary animal care may further complicate an already impaired parent-child relationship marked by child oppositional behavior and parent stress. The time and financial commitment requirements of dog ownership (e.g., training, veterinary care, food) may be more effectively directed toward psychosocial therapies for child and parent (e.g., skills training, parent education). Additionally, there is no guarantee that a particular child-dog relationship will have therapeutic benefit. For behavioral health care providers, a discussion encouraging a careful evaluation of the current state of the family's functionality is crucial; the degree of impairment caused by the child's symptoms across settings, sibling relationships if applicable, marital stress, and parent mental health are all key factors for consideration.

Critical areas for consideration in these circumstances include both child safety and animal welfare. Although the practice of pet ownership in the United States is commonplace, the responsibility of caring for and training an animal with the specific aim of obtaining therapeutic benefit for a child with ADHD is an entirely separate endeavor. In response to these kinds of inquiries, practitioners may instead opt to recommend that prior to pet ownership being pursued, children should participate in a regular animal-assisted activity or intervention with animals specifically trained or selected for these purposes outside of the home. These opportunities may include visitation programs at public libraries or community centers and animal training and education programs at local animal shelters.

Conclusion

The role of dogs in the lives of children with ADHD, both at home and in therapeutic settings, is complex and still not well understood. Although dog ownership in homes with children is commonplace, we know less about the benefits and challenges for families with a child who has ADHD. Emerging evidence suggests that AAIs with dogs are beneficial, but the specific mechanisms by which these benefits result are only speculative at this time. We know little about how individual differences (in dogs and children) and differences in dose or method of intervention may affect benefits and ability to integrate these therapies into existing practices.

Burgeoning evidence, however, supports integrating trained therapy dogs into evidence-based psychosocial interventions for children with ADHD as well as universal programming for students in schools. This growing body of information is especially timely in the current pandemic era as practitioners and educators are faced with significantly increasing rates of mental health challenges among children and adolescents in general, and exponentially greater impairment and comorbid diagnoses in those who had ADHD before the stressors of the pandemic. Therefore, it is paramount that research in this area continues and that practitioners inform themselves about the current evidence and standards of practice when considering the use of AAIs or discussing their use with families.

Resources for Training and Aims for Animal-Assisted Therapy

For clinicians compelled to integrate the assistance of a therapy dog into practice, there are volunteer organizations with nationwide affiliates that provide visits to therapeutic facilities (e.g., https://therapyanimals.org/ita-programs). Several reputable nonprofit organizations in the United States are dedicated to providing registration programs for volunteer handler/animal dyads. Most organizations hold regular trainings for individuals interested in determining if their own pet is a suitable candidate for registration. The American Kennel Club recognizes several organizations that provide certification and registration for dogs formally identified as therapy dogs.

These organizations are important because they aim to set a standard for animal behavior in therapeutic and community settings. Most provide specific training about animal welfare and set limits on animal work and visitations with the aim of protecting the animal from fatigue or risk for abuse, in keeping with the position statements of the American Humane Society and the International Association of Human-Animal Interaction Organizations. It is critical that clinicians seeking to incorporate their own animal into their practice be aware of these standards and guidelines before attempting to integrate animals into their practice with specific therapeutic aims. Practitioners should be mindful that the developing field of AAIs must be continually evaluated, scrutinized, and adjusted across settings and populations, especially with children with special needs and as practices are informed by quality research. A more comprehensive list of resources is provided below.

Standards for therapy dogs	https://petpartners.org https://www.akc.org/products-services/training-programs/canine-good-citizen
Certification programs for therapy dogs	https://socialwork.du.edu/humananimalconnection/education-certificates/animals-human-health-certificate https://petpartners.org/learn/online-education https://www.akc.org/sports/title-recognition-program/therapy-dog-program/therapy-dog-organizations
Position statements	https://www.americanhumane.org/position-statement/therapy-animals https://iahaio.org/position-statements

Key Clinical Points

- Clinicians and health care providers who wish to incorporate animal-assisted interventions (AAIs) or animal-assisted therapy (AAT) in a treatment plan are ethically responsible for developing a background in the area before doing so.

- An AAI treatment program including elements of unstructured child-animal bonding opportunities, structured social skills training, and structured dog-themed activities is indicated for children with ADHD.

- Clinicians and health care providers are urged to establish a clear written protocol for AAI including standards for risk assessment and procedures for safe and humane animal treatment.

- Individual differences in patients and in animals must be carefully considered when determining a treatment plan and accompanying AAI protocol for implementation.

- Clinicians and health care providers incorporating AAI in their practice must stay abreast of topics relevant in the field, including changes in laws, industry guidelines, and insurance policies.

References

Antshel KM: Psychosocial interventions in attention-deficit/hyperactivity disorder: update. Child Adolesc Psychiatr Clin N Am 24(1):79–97, 2015 25455577

Aviv TM, Katz YJ, Berant E: The contribution of therapeutic horseback riding to the improvement of executive functions and self-esteem among children with ADHD. J Atten Disord 25(12):1743–1753, 2021 32508191

Baweja R, Hale DE, Waxmonsky JG: Impact of CNS stimulants for attention-deficit/hyperactivity disorder on growth: epidemiology and approaches to management in children and adolescents. CNS Drugs 35(8):839–859, 2021 34297331

Becker JL, Rogers EC, Burrows B: Animal-assisted social skills training for children with autism spectrum disorders. Anthrozoos 30:307–326, 2017

Bray EE, Gruen ME, Gnanadesikan GE, et al: Cognitive characteristics of 8- to 10-week-old assistance dog puppies. Anim Behav 166:193–206, 2020 32719570

Brelsford VL, Meints K, Gee NR, Pfeffer K: Animal-assisted interventions in the classroom: a systematic review. Int J Environ Res Public Health 14(7):669, 2017 28640200

Cahill L, Prins B, Weber M, McGaugh JL: β-adrenergic activation and memory for emotional events. Nature 371(6499):702–704, 1994 7935815

Carlisle GK: The social skills and attachment to dogs of children with autism spectrum disorder. J Autism Dev Disord 45(5):1137–1145, 2015 25308197

Carucci S, Balia C, Gagliano A, et al: Long term methylphenidate exposure and growth in children and adolescents with ADHD: a systematic review and meta-analysis. Neurosci Biobehav Rev 120:509–525, 2021 33080250

Catalá-López F, Hutton B, Núñez-Beltrán A, et al: The pharmacological and non-pharmacological treatment of attention deficit hyperactivity disorder in children and adolescents: a systematic review with network meta-analyses of randomised trials. PLoS One 12(7):e0180355, 2017 28700715

Caye A, Swanson J, Thapar A, et al: Life span studies of ADHD: conceptual challenges and predictors of persistence and outcome. Curr Psychiatry Rep 18(12):111, 2016 27783340

Caye A, Swanson JM, Coghill D, Rohde LA: Treatment strategies for ADHD: an evidence-based guide to select optimal treatment. Mol Psychiatry 24(3):390–408, 2019 29955166

Childress AC, Komolova M, Sallee FR: An update on the pharmacokinetic considerations in the treatment of ADHD with long-acting methylphenidate and amphetamine formulations. Expert Opin Drug Metab Toxicol 15(11):937–974, 2019 31581854

Concordia Pharmaceuticals: Kapvay® (clonidine hydrochloride) extended-release tablets, for oral use. 2020. Available at: https://www.accessdata.fda.gov/drugsatfda_docs/label/2020/022331s021lbl.pdf. Accessed October 24, 2021.

Cortese S, Adamo N, Del Giovane C, et al: Comparative efficacy and tolerability of medications for attention-deficit hyperactivity disorder in children, adolescents, and adults: a systematic review and network meta-analysis. Lancet Psychiatry 5(9):727–738, 2018 30097390

Crossman MK, Kazdin AE: Additional evidence is needed to recommend acquiring a dog to families of children with autism spectrum disorder: a response to Wright and colleagues. J Autism Dev Disord 46(1):332–335, 2016 26231204

Danielson ML, Visser SN, Gleason MM, et al: A national profile of attention-deficit hyperactivity disorder diagnosis and treatment among US children aged 2 to 5 years. J Dev Behav Pediatr 38(7):455–464, 2017 28723824

Deming J, Jones K, Caldwell S, Phillips A: KIDS: Kids Interacting With Dogs Safely. Englewood, CO, American Humane Association, 2009

Doshi JA, Hodgkins P, Kahle J, et al: Economic impact of childhood and adult attention-deficit/hyperactivity disorder in the United States. J Am Acad Child Adolesc Psychiatry 51(10):990–1002.e2, 2012 23021476

Fabiano GA, Schatz NK, Aloe AM, et al: A systematic review of meta-analyses of psychosocial treatment for attention-deficit/hyperactivity disorder. Clin Child Fam Psychol Rev 18(1):77–97, 2015 25691358

Faraone SV, Sergeant J, Gillberg C, Biederman J: The worldwide prevalence of ADHD: is it an American condition? World Psychiatry 2(2):104–113, 2003 16946911

Flory K, Molina BSG, Pelham WE Jr, et al: Childhood ADHD predicts risky sexual behavior in young adulthood. J Clin Child Adolesc Psychol 35(4):571–577, 2006 17007602

Franke B, Michelini G, Asherson P, et al: Live fast, die young? A review on the developmental trajectories of ADHD across the lifespan. Eur Neuropsychopharmacol 28(10):1059–1088, 2018 30195575

Gee NR, Crist EN, Carr DN: Preschool children require fewer instructional prompts to perform a memory task in the presence of a dog. Anthrozoos 23:173–184, 2010

Gee NR, Fine AH, Schuck S: Animals in educational settings: research and practice, in Handbook on Animal-Assisted Therapy, 4th Edition. Edited by Fine AH. San Diego, CA, Academic Press, 2015, pp 195–210

Gilboa Y, Helmer A: Self-management intervention for attention and executive functions using equine-assisted occupational therapy among children aged 6–14 diagnosed with attention deficit/hyperactivity disorder. J Altern Complement Med 26(3):239–246, 2020 31934771

Green CD, Langberg JM: A review of predictors of psychosocial service utilization in youth with attention-deficit/hyperactivity disorder. Clin Child Fam Psychol Rev 25(2):356–375, 2022 34498154

Hoagwood KE, Acri M, Morrissey M, Peth-Pierce R: Animal-assisted therapies for youth with or at risk for mental health problems: a systematic review. Appl Dev Sci 21(1):1–13, 2017 28798541

Hodgkins P, Shaw M, Coghill D, Hechtman L: Amfetamine and methylphenidate medications for attention-deficit/hyperactivity disorder: complementary treatment options. Eur Child Adolesc Psychiatry 21(9):477–492, 2012 22763750

Howard AL, Kennedy TM, Mitchell JT, et al: Early substance use in the pathway from childhood attention-deficit/hyperactivity disorder (ADHD) to young adult substance use: evidence of statistical mediation and substance specificity. Psychol Addict Behav 34(2):281–292, 2020 31886682

Jones MG, Rice SM, Cotton SM: Incorporating animal-assisted therapy in mental health treatments for adolescents: a systematic review of canine assisted psychotherapy. PLoS One 14(1):e0210761, 2019 30653587

Joseph A, Ayyagari R, Xie M, et al: Comparative efficacy and safety of attention-deficit/hyperactivity disorder pharmacotherapies, including guanfacine extended release: a mixed treatment comparison. Eur Child Adolesc Psychiatry 26(8):875–897, 2017 28258319

Juríčková V, Bozděchová A, Machová K, Vadroňová M: Effect of animal assisted education with a dog within children with ADHD in the classroom: a case study. Child Adolesc Social Work J 37:677–684, 2020

Kotrschal K, Ortbauer B: Behavioral effects of the presence of a dog in a classroom. Anthrozoos 16:147–159, 2003

McGaugh JL: Make mild moments memorable: add a little arousal. Trends Cogn Sci 10(8):345–347, 2006 16793325

Molina BSG, Pelham WE Jr: Childhood predictors of adolescent substance use in a longitudinal study of children with ADHD. J Abnorm Psychol 112(3):497–507, 2003 12943028

MTA Cooperative Group: National Institute of Mental Health Multimodal Treatment Study of ADHD follow-up: changes in effectiveness and growth after the end of treatment. Pediatrics 113(4):762–769, 2004 15060225

O'Haire ME, McKenzie SJ, Beck AM, Slaughter V: Social behaviors increase in children with autism in the presence of animals compared to toys. PLoS One 8(2):e57010, 2013 23468902

Pelham WEJr, Fabiano GA, Waxmonsky JG, et al: Treatment sequencing for childhood ADHD: a multiple-randomization study of adaptive medication and behavioral interventions. J Clin Child Adolesc Psychol 45(4):396–415, 2016 26882332

Rabbitt SM, Kazdin AE, Hong JE: Acceptability of animal-assisted therapy: attitudes toward AAT, psychotherapy, and medication for the treatment of child disruptive behavioral problems. Anthrozoos 27:335–350, 2014

Robb JA, Sibley MH, Pelham WE Jr, et al: The estimated annual cost of ADHD to the U.S. education system. School Ment Health 3(3):169–177, 2011 25110528

Schneider BN, Enenbach M: Managing the risks of ADHD treatments. Curr Psychiatry Rep 16(10):479, 2014 25135779

Schuck SEB, Emmerson NA, Fine AH, et al: Developing the P.A.C.K.: combining canine assisted therapy and cognitive behavioral interventions for children with ADHD. Presented at the poster symposium: Research on Human-Animal Interaction and Youth Socioemotional Development at the Society for Research in Child Development biennial meeting, Seattle, WA, April 18–20, 2013

Schuck SEB, Emmerson NA, Fine AH, Lakes KD: Canine-assisted therapy for children with ADHD: preliminary findings from the Positive Assertive Cooperative Kids study. J Atten Disord 19(2):125–137, 2015 24062278

Schuck SEB, Emmerson NA, Abdullah MM, et al: A randomized controlled trial of traditional psychosocial and canine-assisted intervention for children with ADHD. Hum Anim Interact Bull 6:64–80, 2018a

Schuck SEB, Johnson HL, Abdullah MM, et al: The role of animal assisted intervention on improving self-esteem in children with attention deficit/hyperactivity disorder. Front Pediatr 6:300, 2018b 30450352

Selamat NW, Renganathan Y, Karim SA: Intervention approaches for children with autism spectrum disorder (ASD) and attention hyperactivity disorder

(ADHD): review of research between 2013 and 2017. J Child Adolesc Behav 6:369, 2018

Shire U.S.: Intuniv (guanfacine) extended-release tablets, for oral use. 2019. Available at: https://www.accessdata.fda.gov/drugsatfda_docs/label/2019/022037s019lbl.pdf. Accessed October 17, 2021.

Steingard R, Taskiran S, Connor DF, et al: New formulations of stimulants: an update for clinicians. J Child Adolesc Psychopharmacol 29(5):324–339, 2019 31038360

Takeda Pharmaceuticals: Vyvanse (lisdexamfetamine dimesylate) capsules, for oral use, CII. 2021. Available at: https://www.accessdata.fda.gov/drugsatfda_docs/label/2021/021977s046,208510s003lbl.pdf. Accessed September 18, 2021.

Thompson AL, Molina BSG, Pelham W Jr, Gnagy EM: Risky driving in adolescents and young adults with childhood ADHD. J Pediatr Psychol 32(7):745–759, 2007 17442694

Trampush JW, Miller CJ, Newcorn JH, Halperin JM: The impact of childhood ADHD on dropping out of high school in urban adolescents/young adults. J Atten Disord 13(2):127–136, 2009 18757845

Valley-Damkoehler DA: Animal-Assisted Therapy and Attention-Deficit Hyperactivity Disorder Youth Program: A Grant Proposal. Long Beach, California State University, 2019

Wells KC, Pelham WE, Kotkin RA, et al: Psychosocial treatment strategies in the MTA study: rationale, methods, and critical issues in design and implementation. J Abnorm Child Psychol 28(6):483–505, 2000 11104313

Wolraich ML, Chan E, Froehlich T, et al: ADHD diagnosis and treatment guidelines: a historical perspective. Pediatrics 144(4):e20191682, 2019 31570649

Yerkes RM, Dodson JD: The relation of strength of stimulus to rapidity of habit-formation. J Comp Neurol Psychol 18(5):27–41, 1908

7

Companion Animals in the Treatment of Autism Spectrum Disorder

Marguerite E. O'Haire, Ph.D.
Kerri E. Rodriguez, Ph.D.
Leanne O. Nieforth, Ph.D.
Alice R. Mao, M.D.

AUTISM SPECTRUM DISORDER (ASD) is an umbrella term for complex, life-long developmental disorders characterized by persistent deficits in social communication and social interactions as well as restricted, repetitive patterns of behavior. Symptoms of ASD are present in the early developmental period and cause clinically significant impairments in daily functioning. An ASD diagnosis can co-occur with intellectual impairment; language impairment; known medical or genetic conditions; or other associated neurodevelopmental, mental, or behavioral disorders.

Prevalence of Autism Spectrum Disorder and Risk Factors

An estimated 1 in 54 children in the United States currently has ASD, a prevalence that has increased dramatically over the past three decades (Maenner et al. 2020). Global estimates suggest that 1%–2% of the population has ASD (Elsabbagh et al. 2012). Although ASD is 4.3 times more prevalent among boys than among girls, ASD occurs equally in all race/ethnicity and socioeconomic groups (Maenner et al. 2020).

The etiology of and underlying risk factors for ASD are unknown. However, autism rates in twins and within families suggest that autism is highly heritable (Sandin et al. 2014). When one identical twin has ASD, there is a 64%–91% chance that the other twin also has ASD (Tick et al. 2016). However, genetics is not the sole explanatory factor in ASD etiology; twin studies suggest that environmental factors are also important for understanding the etiology of ASD (Hallmayer et al. 2011). Some examples of known environmental risk factors for ASD include prenatal factors (e.g., maternal age, maternal medication use, gestational diabetes), perinatal factors (e.g., cesarean delivery, fetal or umbilical cord complications, gestational age < 36 weeks), and postnatal factors (Gardener et al. 2009).

Clinical Presentation and Longitudinal Time Course

For the diagnostic criteria for ASD to be met, a child must show persistent, clinically significant impairments in social communication and interaction, including deficits in social-emotional reciprocity, deficits in communicative behavior, and deficits in forming and maintaining relationships (American Psychiatric Association 2022). In addition, a child must have restricted, repetitive patterns of behavior, interests, or activities, including stereotyped or repetitive motor movements, insistence on sameness, restricted and fixated interests, and hyper- or hyporeactivity to sensory input.

As the name implies, ASD exists on a "spectrum" because of the wide variation in symptom presentation and severity. Therefore, because of the broad range of symptoms, specifiers, and co-occurring conditions that result in heterogeneous developmental pathways, diagnosing and treating ASD is often complex and challenging (Masi et al. 2017). ASD symptoms must be present in early childhood, even if they are not diagnosed or recognized until later childhood. Although diagnoses can be made reliably by age 2 years (Johnson et al. 2007), most diagnoses do not occur until after age 5 years (Shattuck et al. 2009).

Overview of Existing Evidence-Based Treatments

Early and accurate diagnosis of ASD is extremely beneficial because it allows for effective early intervention. Early interventions that occur at or before preschool age, when the brain is in an optimal state of plasticity, can result in sustained improvements to social, behavioral, and functional impairments (Eldevik et al. 2009). Because of the importance of early intervention in improving short-term and long-term outcomes (see, e.g., Estes et al. 2015), guidelines recommend initiating interventions as soon as possible after diagnosis (Zwaigenbaum et al. 2015). Early behavioral interventions are largely based on applied behavior analysis, which aims to improve social behavior and learning skills through positive reinforcement. Other behavior and communication approaches used to assist in ASD treatment include speech and occupational therapy, social skills training, and the use of assistive technologies to teach communication skills (Masi et al. 2017).

Behavioral interventions may be challenging if a child with ASD has disruptive or maladaptive behaviors such as impulsive aggression, irritability, or self-injury. For these children, medications can also help ameliorate behavioral and mental health symptoms (Becerra et al. 2017). Although no pharmacological treatments are approved by the FDA for the core symptoms of ASD, there is increasing evidence for the pharmacological management of behavioral symptoms associated with ASD, such as irritability and hyperactivity. For example, the atypical antipsychotics risperidone and aripiprazole are FDA approved in the United States for the treatment of irritability associated with ASD (Elbe and Lalani 2012). The antipsychotic olanzapine also has been shown to improve symptoms of irritability and hyperactivity (Hesapcioglu et al. 2020). In addition to antipsychotics, anticonvulsants have been studied as an alternative for management of irritability and aggression in youth with ASD (e.g., Hollander et al. 2010). Finally, although not FDA approved, stimulants such as methylphenidate and selective norepinephrine reuptake inhibitors such as atomoxetine can be effective for the management of hyperactivity and aggression in children with ASD with comorbid ADHD (Joshi et al. 2021). α_2-Antagonists, such as guanfacine and clonidine, also have been used to treat ADHD symptoms in children with autism who were not able to tolerate stimulant medications (Handen et al. 2015).

In addition to behavioral and pharmacological interventions, various complementary and integrative interventions are available for ASD. These practices are used alongside conventional, evidence-based treatments for ASD to address child symptomatology and quality of life. Parents of children with ASD engage in many complementary interventions for their children to address specific impairments and symptoms (Goin-Kochel et al. 2007). A 2010 study found that more than 70% of parents surveyed had tried at least one complementary or alternative intervention for their child, with about 50% currently engaging in one or more of these interventions. Complementary interventions include dietary interventions (e.g., gluten-free or casein-free), nutritional supplementation, and nonbiological interventions such as music therapy, mind-body therapies, and animal-assisted interventions (AAIs) (Hall and Riccio 2012).

Animal-Assisted Interventions

AAIs are goal-oriented interventions that intentionally incorporate animals for the purpose of therapeutic gains in humans (International Association of Human-Animal Interaction Organizations 2018). AAIs contain three subcategories:

1. Animal-assisted therapy (AAT), which involves planned, structured interactions with an animal as part of a therapeutic intervention directed and/or delivered by a health and human services professional
2. Animal-assisted activities (AAAs), which involve informal interaction and visitation by a human-animal team for motivational, educational, and recreational purposes
3. Animal-assisted education, which involves planned, structured interaction with an animal directed and/or delivered by educational professionals

Both AAT and AAAs are common complementary interventions for ASD (Christon et al. 2010). In addition to these short-term, goal-oriented interactions with animals, individuals with ASD may benefit from the long-term placement of an autism service dog in the home. Autism service dogs are a type of psychiatric service dog who is trained to perform tasks aimed to mitigate ASD symptoms and improve well-being.

One of the original theoretical explanations underlying positive human-animal interactions is the biophilia hypothesis, which states that animals may act as a positive external focus of attention (Wilson 1984). This focus on the animal may serve to subsequently enhance concentration, reduce distraction, and limit anxious arousal for individuals with ASD (Kruger and Serpell 2010; Melson 2000). In one of the first published observations of AAT for children with ASD, it was proposed that the animal's sensory and perceptual appeal helped facilitate therapist interaction, resulting in fewer repetitive behaviors (e.g., hand-flapping, jumping) and more socially appropriate behavior toward the therapist (Redefer and Goodman 1989). A widely supported theory of human-animal interaction, social support theory, states that animals act as a nonjudgmental source of support and a catalyst for social interaction (McNicholas and Collis 2006). In this regard, animals may help individuals with ASD initiate verbal social interaction and maintain positive social behavior with peers, caregivers, and therapy professionals (Martin and Farnum 2002).

The biopsychosocial model is another proposed theory describing how therapeutic mechanisms are interrelated across the three influencers of health (i.e., biological, psychological, and social; Gee et al. 2021). Positive psychosocial effects of animal interaction are linked with positive biological effects (e.g., decreased heart rate, blood pressure, and cortisol; increased oxytocin) (Beetz et al. 2012). In this context, animal interaction may confer both psychosocial and physiological benefits for individuals with ASD in an interrelated and dynamic manner. Taken together, current theories of human-animal interaction suggest meaningful pathways for animal interaction to confer unique benefits for individuals with ASD.

Scientific Evidence Base

To synthesize the current research on AAI for ASD, we compiled findings from three comprehensive systematic reviews inclusively spanning the period from 1989 to 2020 (Nieforth et al. 2021; O'Haire 2017; O'Haire et al. 2015). Findings were aggregated across 85 peer-reviewed scientific publications to identify the trajectory of the field over time, the global reach of the findings, and the key characteristics of the samples and outcomes. The number of studies on the effects of AAIs for ASD is relatively high compared with the number of studies on AAI for other psychiatric diagnoses (see, e.g., Hoagwood et al. 2017), indicating a strong interest in studying outcomes for this population.

Growth of the Field

The number of peer-reviewed studies on AAIs for ASD has increased over time (Figure 7–1). Most of this research (87%) has occurred within

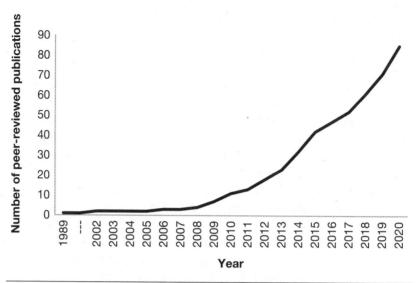

Figure 7–1. **Number of peer-reviewed scientific publications on animal-assisted interventions for autism spectrum disorder from 1989 to 2020.**

the past decade (2011–2020). More than half (51%) of the publications in the entire field of research appeared between 2016 and 2020. This growth indicates an increasing interest and focus on the provision of AAIs as a complementary intervention modality for individuals with ASD.

International Representation

Among publications written in English, there is a broad international representation of research teams (Figure 7–2). The largest portion of studies emerged from North America (44%) and Europe (34%). However, research teams studying AAIs for ASD were also located in Asia, Australia, South America, and Africa. This worldwide spread of investigators substantiates the topic's global relevance.

Intervention Characteristics

Animal Participants

A broad range of species have been evaluated in research on AAIs for ASD (Figure 7–3). The most common species were horses (42%) and

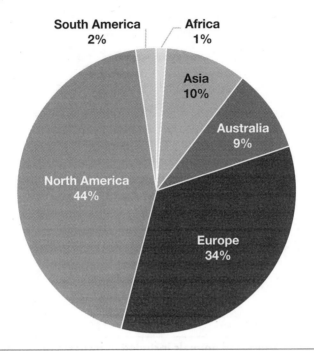

Figure 7–2. Continents of lead authors on peer-reviewed scientific publications on animal-assisted interventions for autism spectrum disorder.

dogs (36%). Other studies examined outcomes from AAIs with a combination of more than one species (e.g., farm animals), guinea pigs, or dolphins. Little research has been done on AAIs with cats; we found only one study with cats as the sole AAI animal. Given the preponderance of data on horses and dogs (nearly 79% together), most research findings to date are related to those species.

Human Participants

Interventions involving AAIs for ASD are primarily conducted with children, not teenagers or adults. The average age of participants in the studies was between 9 and 10 years. The gender breakdown is primarily male (approximately 80%), which aligns with diagnostic frequency among males versus females of ASD. Few studies reported on race/ethnicity; therefore, it is largely unknown whether there are any differential effects across race/ethnicity.

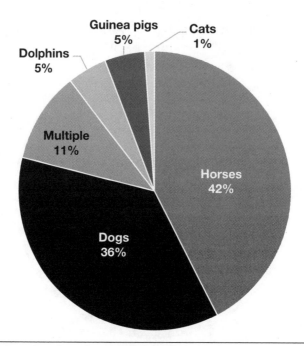

Figure 7–3.   Species of animals included in research on animal-assisted interventions for autism spectrum disorder.

Intervention Activities

The activities involved in AAIs are wide-ranging, often with minimal description and a lack of manualized programs. There is a growing movement to develop standards and replicable programs of AAIs for ASD, yet it is currently unknown which activities are most efficacious (see, e.g., O'Haire 2017). The core feature of these programs is often the presence of an animal during typical treatment sessions or enrichment activities centering around interacting with or caring for the animal. Intervention sessions are typically conducted on a weekly basis for 30–60 minutes, with an average dose of approximately 10 hours of contact time with the animals over the course of an AAI program.

Outcomes of Animal-Assisted Interventions for Autism Spectrum Disorder

Across 85 studies on AAIs for ASD, a range of socioemotional outcomes were assessed. Ten key finding categories were synthesized to represent

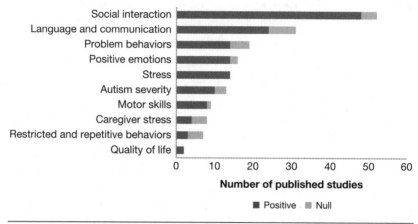

Figure 7–4. **Number of studies assessing and reporting positive and null outcomes from animal-assisted interventions for autism spectrum disorder.**

the most prevalent outcomes in research studies (Figure 7–4). Although findings were predominantly positive, a subset of findings in each category were null, wherein no significant difference was found following the AAI. Null findings are important to recognize in order to understand the variability of outcomes and to acknowledge that not all children and animals will respond uniformly (Rodriguez et al. 2021). Not all outcomes can be expected for every child, and providers should sensitively assess (and reassess) the appropriateness and efficacy of an AAI for each individual with ASD over time.

Social Interaction

The most common outcome of AAIs for ASD was increased social interaction (Nieforth et al. 2021). The robustness of this effect is evidenced by its replication across different researchers around the globe. Positive findings for social interaction in individuals with ASD have been reported in 48 studies by 40 research teams across 19 countries (Nieforth et al. 2021; O'Haire 2017; O'Haire et al. 2015).

Findings include increases in both the frequency and the quality of social interactions. Examples include increased talking, smiling, and looking at human faces in the presence of an animal. Social responsiveness and empathy are also cited as enhancing social interactions. The ways in which animals motivated social interaction included improvements in joint attention, overall social skills, and general social functioning. Importantly, animal interaction was found to improve social interaction with both child peers and adult caregivers and professionals.

Communication, Emotions, and Stress

Related to social interactions, the second most frequent outcome of AAIs for ASD was increased language and communication (Nieforth et al. 2021; O'Haire 2017; O'Haire et al. 2015). Most studies reported increases in both receptive and expressive language, although a subset of studies found no changes. Some children with ASD had a change in overall demeanor as well, with reductions in challenging behaviors and increases in positive emotions. If the animal's presence elicits more effective communication and social interaction, then challenging behaviors may be less of an outlet for communication. Indeed, some studies also showed reductions in stress, assessed both subjectively and physiologically via the stress hormone cortisol. Emerging literature is beginning to evaluate the effect of AAIs on the stress of not only the individual with ASD but also their parents or caregivers. Findings in this domain have been mixed, particularly for caregivers who are responsible for the animal as well as the child, which may increase caregiver burden. Taken together, initial findings are most promising for enhanced social interactions for the child and the domains that flow on from these gains such as increased communication and emotional well-being.

Strength and Quality of the Evidence Base

Although there are a growing number of studies on AAIs for ASD, several limitations restrict our understanding of outcomes. First, there are few randomized clinical trials, which are the gold standard for evaluating treatment efficacy. Second, the findings are largely based on parent-reported outcomes rather than outcomes reported by masked observers or clinicians. The insight from parents is critical, because they are the key individuals familiar with the child's behavior and, most importantly, are affected by the child's behavior. However, additional respondents and assessment modalities will strengthen our understanding of nuanced and objective outcomes.

Third, ASD is a spectrum disorder with broad heterogeneity, yet little research is available on the mediators and moderators of treatment outcomes. In other words, we do not yet have informative data on which clients will most likely benefit from a given intervention and under what circumstances. It is currently unknown whether one species is superior to another, what the most effective or required dosage of animal interaction is, and which intervention activities or strategies are most effective. In addition, few studies have evaluated the elements or components that drive outcomes. There has been some criticism that without further studies using active, attention control conditions, it is hard to know if the observed benefits of AAIs are due to the novelty of the intervention or to the animal specifically.

Finally, in areas with the potential for placebo effects or expectancy biases such as human-animal interaction research, there is often the risk of a "file drawer" effect. Specifically, positive findings may be more likely to be published, whereas null or negative findings are often "filed away" unpublished. The findings in this chapter are summarized from peer-reviewed, published journal articles rather than from unpublished sources such as dissertations and conference presentations. Thus, there is a risk that this synthesis overestimates positive outcomes. These limitations should be taken into account when one is interpreting the outcomes from existing published research.

Clinical Practice Implications

The current literature suggests that AAIs for ASD may be effective, and future exploration is warranted. An analysis of the methodological rigor of studies suggests that the current evidence base is limited by methodological flaws and a lack of randomized controlled trial designs. Therefore, caution should be exercised in selecting an AAI as a complementary intervention for ASD. As with the selection of any intervention, the needs of the specific client should be at the forefront of the decision. We suggest consulting with the client, the client's family, and the client's larger care team to determine the best possible course of action for all individuals involved. Clinicians may need to field questions related to acquiring a companion animal (e.g., horse or dog) for the individual. We recommend that clinicians educate families about the differences between a companion animal and an AAI. Educating families on the differences will help to clarify the goals that the families have and will help determine the best course of action for the particular individual. The literature thus far has focused on AAI for ASD and is inconclusive regarding companion animals and ASD. We encourage clinicians to speak openly about the pros and cons of these interventions in order to create a more well-rounded expectation for the client and their family. When

Table 7–1. **Client characteristics to consider in determining whether an animal-assisted intervention would be useful**

Client characteristic	Example
Current treatment	If a client is taking a medication that may negatively influence balance because of its sedating effects, walking a dog on a leash may not be the best activity choice during animal-assisted intervention.
Age	Children younger than 2 years should not participate in mounted equine-assisted services because they are not yet physically or neurologically developed enough to withstand movement from the horse's gait. Children younger than 5 years may not have the motor control necessary to carefully interact with small animals, such as guinea pigs.
Sensory impairment	If a client is easily or severely overwhelmed by sensory stimulation, it may be better for them to participate in more passive types of interventions (e.g., watching a herd of horses interact in a large pasture) rather than physically interacting with animals (e.g., dog walking, horseback riding).
Mobility impairment	If a client has a mobility impairment in which riding a horse would cause pain, riding during equine-assisted services would not be the correct option, but interacting with the horse on the ground could be an appropriate alternative.

clinicians are determining whether an AAI would be useful for a particular client, we recommend addressing the following considerations.

Who Is the Client?

Client characteristics to consider are listed in Table 7–1.

Does the Client Have Any Contraindications to Taking Part in Animal-Assisted Interventions?

The safety of the client, animal, and practitioners in AAIs is paramount. With this in mind, a few contraindications to participation should be

Table 7–2. Contraindications to participation to consider when determining whether an animal-assisted intervention (AAI) would be beneficial for a client

Contraindication	Example
Fear of animals	If a client fears animals, it would be unethical to force them to participate in an AAI session unless that fear can be safely mitigated.
Behavior challenges that result in harm to people	In an equine-assisted intervention session, three volunteers typically work with the client (one on each side of the horse and another leading the horse). These volunteers ensure the safety of the client and the horse. If the client were to engage in aggressive behavior during the session, they would endanger themselves, the volunteers, and the horse.
Behavior challenges that result in harm to animals	If a client has indicated a desire to harm animals or shown aggressive or harmful behavior toward an animal in the past, it is contraindicated for that client to participate.
Allergy to animals or something in the AAI environment	An allergy to animals, hay, or grass would be a contraindication to use of equine-assisted services.
Immunocompromised status	Any interaction with an animal brings with it the possibility of zoonotic disease exposure.

considered when determining whether an AAI would be beneficial for a client (Table 7–2).

What Do You Hope the Client Will Gain From Participating in Animal-Assisted Interventions?

Studies suggest that AAIs are most effective for improving communication and social skills for participants with ASD (Nieforth et al. 2021). The influence of AAIs on ASD severity and problem behaviors is less well known because findings are mixed. In weighing options for AAI programs, selecting the program best suited for achieving a particular outcome for the client is important. Few studies have quantified long-term outcomes of AAI, but benefits apparent during or directly after AAIs may not be maintained after the intervention is removed. AAIs may be most effective when offered to the client routinely.

What Animal-Assisted Interventions Are Available to the Client?

The variation of AAIs for ASD should be taken into consideration in determining the best course of action for a particular client. One source of variation lies in the training of interventionists. Some interventionists have completed advanced academic training (master's or Ph.D. level), whereas others have completed industry trainings and certifications. Among equine-assisted services certifications, the most common is the Professional Association of Therapeutic Horsemanship (PATH). Most of the current research on equine-assisted services for ASD takes place at a PATH-accredited facility or emulates the PATH model with its structure. Training for other types of AAIs is less uniform, with multiple programs and certifications available for handlers.

Another source of variation lies in the role and training of therapy animals. No standardized specific training model is available for any species involved in AAIs. Each certification and program has different temperament, behavior, health, and training requirements for therapy animals. Most animals are selected on the basis of having the appropriate temperament and behavior when working with a particular population of clients. Selecting a program that puts human and animal welfare at the forefront of the intervention is crucial.

The third source of variation lies in the intervention itself. This variation is apparent in the setting of the intervention (e.g., client's home, practitioner's office, school, horse farm), the length of a session (ranging from 15 minutes to multiple hours), the activities engaged in (interacting with the animal vs. coexisting with the animal), and the ratio of participants to interventionists (dependent on species and program).

There is a great need for standardization of treatment strategies, outcome measures, and collection of data among different types of AAIs. Until types of AAIs for ASD are standardized, it is important to fully understand the AAI programs available to clients to make the most accurate referral. Although variation in AAIs exists across the industry, referrals should be based on selecting a locally available, high-quality intervention.

What Might an Animal-Assisted Intervention Session Look Like?

AAI sessions can be individualized to each client in terms of the species chosen for the intervention and in terms of the activities or interactions with the animal. Tables 7–3, 7–4, and 7–5 highlight three example skills that can be developed with AAIs across three different species.

Table 7–3.   Example skill #1: building empathy

Dog	Horse	Guinea pig
While sitting next to and petting the dog, ask the client: How does the dog feel when you pet her? How do you know when and where she likes to be petted? How can you make her feel happy or calm?	While grooming the horse, ask the client: How does the horse feel when he is being brushed? How do you know when the horse feels calm? How can you make him feel happy or calm?	While near the guinea pig, ask the client: How does the guinea pig feel when a person approaches? How do you know when the guinea pig is happy? How can you make him feel happier?

Table 7–4.   Example skill #2: building self-regulation and anxiety reduction skills

Dog	Horse	Guinea pig
Lead the dog through an obstacle course. It is helpful to have multiple levels of difficulty throughout the course. If you get frustrated at a difficult obstacle, tell the dog about your frustration and share what you think the dog is feeling. Once you have finished processing the frustration, move on within the obstacle course.	Stand next to the horse and try to breathe with the horse. Are you breathing faster or slower than the horse? Do you think that the horse is relaxed? Are you relaxed? Lead the horse at a rhythmic walk or trot. When do you feel the horse get out of rhythm? When do you get out of rhythm? Can you walk or trot to the beat of your favorite song?	Sit calmly and take deep breaths while holding the guinea pig. Watch the guinea pig's behavior to determine whether the guinea pig also relaxes. It is a good sign when the guinea pig eats, because this indicates that they are feeling calm. This can provide a visual feedback system to reinforce calming breathing.

Table 7–5.   Example skill #3: building collaboration and social skills

Dog	Horse	Guinea pig
Take the dog on a walk and introduce the dog to three people along the way. Share three facts about the dog when you introduce them. Can you gather one fact about each individual you meet along the way? The people being introduced to the dog can be staff members, other clients (if in a group), or parents/ caregivers of the clients.	In a small riding arena, place two barrels apart from each other (distance depends on skill level). On one barrel have a pile of stuffed horses, and on the other barrel have some grass or hay. Riders communicate to their horse leader (or side walker) which stuffed horse to hand to them. Then the client holds the stuffed horse while riding over to the second barrel to place it in the hay. Not only does the client have to communicate with the volunteer, but they also need to communicate with their horse in telling it to walk and halt to move from one barrel to another.	Work together with your peers to build a tunnel (or house) for the guinea pig with craft supplies. Talk as a group about which materials the guinea pigs might like and how you will put the pieces together. Use opportunities to share materials, discuss plans, and get creative. Another collaborative activity can include preparing food for and feeding the guinea pigs. Provide fresh vegetables that can be broken into smaller pieces. One child can feed while another prepares, and then they can switch. The children may also create a "restaurant" for the guinea pigs and present foods on small plates or in courses.

Key Clinical Points

- When the clinician is determining whether animal-assisted interventions (AAIs) may be appropriate for a specific client, current treatment, age, sensory impairment, and mobility impairment must factor into the evaluation.

- The clinician also must determine whether the client has any contraindications to AAIs, such as fear of animals, behaviors that could result in harm to people or animals, allergies to animals or an animal environment, or an immunocompromised status.

- After determining appropriateness and considering contraindications, the clinician must anticipate what an AAI session designed to work on specific skills might look like.

- After achieving an understanding of what might be gained for the client from participating in an AAI, the clinician can select an appropriate AAI program.

- Finally, the clinician should investigate the quality and availability of suitable AAI programs before deciding on one.

References

American Psychiatric Association: Diagnostic and Statistical Manual of Mental Disorders, 5th Edition, Text Revision. Washington, DC, American Psychiatric Association, 2022

Becerra TA, Massolo ML, Yau VM, et al: A survey of parents with children on the autism spectrum: experience with services and treatments. Perm J 21:16-009, 2017 28488981

Beetz A, Uvnäs-Moberg K, Julius H, Kotrschal K: Psychosocial and psychophysiological effects of human-animal interactions: the possible role of oxytocin. Front Psychol 3:234, 2012 22866043

Christon LM, Mackintosh VH, Myers BJ: Use of complementary and alternative medicine (CAM) treatments by parents of children with autism spectrum disorders. Res Autism Spectr Disord 4(2):249–259, 2010

Elbe D, Lalani Z: Review of the pharmacotherapy of irritability of autism. J Can Acad Child Adolesc Psychiatry 21(2):130–146, 2012 22548111

Eldevik S, Hastings RP, Hughes JC, et al: Meta-analysis of early intensive behavioral intervention for children with autism. J Clin Child Adolesc Psychol
38(3):439–450, 2009 19437303

Elsabbagh M, Divan G, Koh YJ, et al: Global prevalence of autism and other pervasive developmental disorders. Autism Res 5(3):160–179, 2012 22495912

Estes A, Munson J, Rogers SJ, et al: Long-term outcomes of early intervention
in 6-year-old children with autism spectrum disorder. J Am Acad Child Adolesc Psychiatry 54(7):580–587, 2015 26088663

Gardener H, Spiegelman D, Buka SL: Prenatal risk factors for autism: comprehensive meta-analysis. Br J Psychiatry 195(1):7–14, 2009 19567888

Gee NR, Rodriguez KE, Fine AH, Trammell JP: Dogs supporting human health
and well-being: a biopsychosocial approach. Front Vet Sci 8:630465, 2021
33860004

Goin-Kochel RP, Myers BJ, Mackintosh VH: Parental reports on the use of treatments and therapies for children with autism spectrum disorders. Res Autism Spectr Disord 1(3):195–209, 2007

Hall SE, Riccio CA: Complementary and alternative treatment use for autism spectrum disorders. Complement Ther Clin Pract 18(3):159–163, 2012 22789791

Hallmayer J, Cleveland S, Torres A, et al: Genetic heritability and shared environmental factors among twin pairs with autism. Arch Gen Psychiatry
68(11):1095–1102, 2011 21727249

Handen BL, Aman MG, Arnold LE, et al: Atomoxetine, parent training, and their
combination in children with autism spectrum disorder and attention-
deficit/hyperactivity disorder. J Am Acad Child Adolesc Psychiatry
54(11):905–915, 2015 26506581

Hesapcioglu ST, Ceylan MF, Kasak M, Sen CP: Olanzapine, risperidone, and aripiprazole use in children and adolescents with autism spectrum disorders.
Res Autism Spectr Disord 72:101520, 2020

Hoagwood KE, Acri M, Morrissey M, Peth-Pierce R: Animal-assisted therapies
for youth with or at risk for mental health problems: a systematic review.
Appl Dev Sci 21(1):1–13, 2017 28798541

Hollander E, Chaplin W, Soorya L, et al: Divalproex sodium vs placebo for the
treatment of irritability in children and adolescents with autism spectrum
disorders. Neuropsychopharmacology 35(4):990–998, 2010 20010551

International Association of Human-Animal Interaction Organizations: The
IAHAIO Definitions for Animal Assisted Intervention and Guidelines for
Wellness of Animals Involved in AAI. Seattle, WA, IAHAIO, 2018. Available
at: https://iahaio.org/best-practice/white-paper-on-animal-assisted-
interventions. Accessed April 11, 2018.

Johnson CP, Myers SM, American Academy of Pediatrics Council on Children
With Disabilities: Identification and evaluation of children with autism spectrum disorders. Pediatrics 120(5):1183–1215, 2007 17967920

Joshi G, Wilens T, Firmin ES, et al: Pharmacotherapy of attention deficit/hyper-
activity disorder in individuals with autism spectrum disorder: a systematic
review of the literature. J Psychopharmacol 35(3):203–210, 2021 33349107

Kruger KA, Serpell JA: Animal-assisted interventions in mental health: definitions and theoretical foundations, in Handbook on Animal-Assisted Therapy: Theoretical Foundations and Guidelines for Practice, 3rd Edition. Edited by Fine A. San Diego, CA, Academic Press, 2010, pp 33–48

Maenner MJ, Shaw KA, Baio J, et al: Prevalence of autism spectrum disorder among children aged 8 years—Autism and Developmental Disabilities Monitoring Network, 11 sites, United States, 2016. MMWR Surveill Summ 69(4):1–12, 2020 32214087

Martin F, Farnum J: Animal-assisted therapy for children with pervasive developmental disorders. West J Nurs Res 24(6):657–670, 2002 12365766

Masi A, DeMayo MM, Glozier N, Guastella AJ: An overview of autism spectrum disorder, heterogeneity and treatment options. Neurosci Bull 33(2):183–193, 2017 28213805

McNicholas J, Collis GM: Animals as social supports: insights for understanding animal-assisted therapy, in Handbook on Animal-Assisted Therapy: Theoretical Foundations and Guidelines for Practice, 2nd Edition. Edited by Fine A. San Diego, CA, Academic Press, 2006, pp 49–72

Melson GF: Companion animals and the development of children: implications of the biophilia hypothesis, in Handbook on Animal-Assisted Therapy: Theoretical Foundations and Guidelines for Practice. Edited by Fine A. San Diego, CA, Academic Press, 2000, pp 375–383

Nieforth LO, Schwichtenberg AJ, O'Haire ME: Animal-assisted interventions for autism spectrum disorder: a systematic review of the literature from 2016 to 2020. Rev J Autism Dev Disord 30:1–26, 2021

O'Haire ME: Research on animal-assisted intervention and autism spectrum disorder, 2012–2015. Appl Dev Sci 21(3):200–216, 2017 31080343

O'Haire ME, Guérin NA, Kirkham AC: Animal-assisted intervention for trauma: a systematic literature review. Front Psychol 6:1121, 2015 26300817

Redefer LA, Goodman JF: Brief report: pet-facilitated therapy with autistic children. J Autism Dev Disord 19(3):461–467, 1989 2793790

Rodriguez KE, Herzog H, Gee NR: Variability in human-animal interaction research. Front Vet Sci 7:619600, 2021 33521092

Sandin S, Lichtenstein P, Kuja-Halkola R, et al: The familial risk of autism. JAMA 311(17):1770–1777, 2014 24794370

Shattuck PT, Durkin M, Maenner M, et al: Timing of identification among children with an autism spectrum disorder: findings from a population-based surveillance study. J Am Acad Child Adolesc Psychiatry 48(5):474–483, 2009 19318992

Tick B, Bolton P, Happé F, et al: Heritability of autism spectrum disorders: a meta-analysis of twin studies. J Child Psychol Psychiatry 57(5):585–595, 2016 26709141

Wilson EO: Biophilia. Cambridge, MA, Harvard University Press, 1984

Zwaigenbaum L, Bauman ML, Choueiri R, et al: Early intervention for children with autism spectrum disorder under 3 years of age: recommendations for practice and research. Pediatrics 136(Suppl 1):S60–S81, 2015 26430170

8

Companion Animals in the Treatment of Depressive Disorders

Lisa D. Townsend, Ph.D., LCSW
Nancy R. Gee, Ph.D.
Susan G. Kornstein, M.D.

WE DESCRIBE THE role of animal-assisted interventions (AAIs), animal-assisted therapies (AATs), and companion animals (pets) as adjunctive treatments to evidence-based strategies for treating depression. We discuss potential mechanisms of effect for AAIs and AATs as well as specific populations for whom such treatments show promise.

Prevalence of Depressive Disorders and Risk Factors

Major depressive disorder (MDD) represents one of the most common and debilitating illnesses and affects millions of people across the globe. In the United States, 10% of adults have experienced a major depressive episode in the past year, and 21% have experienced one in their lifetime; the rates are about twice as high in women as in men (Hasin et al. 2018).

Depression can strike at any time throughout the life course, with a heightened risk window beginning in adolescence and extending into early adulthood (Rohde et al. 2009). Well-known risk factors for depression include female sex, being unmarried or without a long-term partner, and younger age (Kessler and Bromet 2013), as well as childbearing (Wisner et al. 2013), chronic medical illness (Katon 2003), and childhood adversity (Giano et al. 2021).

Clinical Presentation and Longitudinal Time Course

Hallmark symptoms of depression include persistently low mood (alternatively, irritability in children and adolescents) and loss of interest or pleasure in all or nearly all activities (American Psychiatric Association 2022) for at least 2 weeks, along with an array of features such as sleep and appetite changes, fatigue or decreased energy, concentration difficulties, feelings of guilt or worthlessness, and thoughts of death or suicide. Depressive disorders interfere with critical milestones across the life course such as education completion (Kessler et al. 1995), employment (Merikangas et al. 2007), and relationship stability (Mojtabai et al. 2017). Poorly controlled depression exacerbates the morbidity of chronic physical illnesses (Moussavi et al. 2007) and costs billions of dollars each year in personal and occupational losses (Wang et al. 2003). Of critical concern, depression is a significant risk factor for suicidal ideation and suicide attempt (Nock et al. 2009) as well as completed suicide (Harris and Barraclough 1997).

Overview of Evidence-Based Treatment of Depression

Current gold-standard treatment of depression involves psychotherapy, medication, or a combination of both. American Psychological Association (2019) psychotherapy practice guidelines recommend cognitive-behavioral-based modalities in addition to interpersonal, psychodynamic, and supportive therapies for depressed adults. The same guidelines suggest cognitive-behavioral therapy (CBT) or interpersonal psychotherapy for depressed adolescents. Group CBT or life review interventions are emphasized for older adults with depression. Although these interventions are often efficacious on their own, depressive disorders associated with severe impairment or suicidal ideation often warrant the addition of pharmacotherapeutic agents.

There are several different classes of antidepressant medications. The most commonly used are selective serotonin reuptake inhibitors, such as fluoxetine and sertraline; serotonin-norepinephrine reuptake inhibitors, such as venlafaxine and duloxetine; and atypical antidepressants, such as bupropion and mirtazapine. Antidepressants generally take 1–2 months to reach their full benefit. The duration of antidepressant treatment needed for a single episode of depression is 6–12 months, but long-term treatment is required for patients with a recurrent course of illness. Many patients will require several trials or a combination of different agents to achieve remission.

Although many patients achieve depression remission with psychotherapy, pharmacotherapy, or both, some individuals struggle with failure to respond to treatment, relapse, or recurrence. In addition, some people may experience difficulty engaging in psychotherapy or hesitance to take medications. For these populations, the involvement of animals may augment treatment effects by acting on primary symptoms themselves or improving the therapeutic process through enhanced engagement and reduced attrition (Jones et al. 2019).

Role of Animals in Depression Treatment

Ways of Involving Animals in Treatment

Equines and canines are the most common animals to play a role in the treatment of depressive disorders. Equine-assisted interventions and therapies are typically guided by the Equine Assisted Growth and Learning Association (www.eagala.org) and the Professional Association of Therapeutic Horsemanship International (www.pathintl.org) models and involve activities such as grooming and feeding horses, walking them on a lead, guiding them through an obstacle course, observing their responses to human behavior, and sometimes riding them. Canine-assisted activities range from the simple presence of a dog to petting, grooming, feeding, training, and walking activities. Canine-assisted interventions can be conducted in a variety of ways, ranging from dog visitation, in which a registered therapy dog visits in a hospital or other treatment setting, to formalized interventions in group or individual therapy sessions. Activities can be unstructured, arising organically between the patient and the dog, or highly structured, such as involving a therapy dog in a CBT session to facilitate skill acquisition.

Therapeutic modalities can be undergirded by cognitive-behavioral, solution-focused, motivational-enhancement, or supportive psychotherapy theories, among other approaches. Interventions can be individual- or group-based, depending on the treatment goals and setting. Whether an animal-assisted activity is characterized as an intervention or as a therapy depends on the training of those who are conducting the session and whether specific treatment goals are formalized and measured. AATs require the presence of a licensed mental health professional and documentation of treatment strategies and patient outcomes, whereas AAIs can be conducted by nonlicensed handlers for therapeutic purposes (International Association of Human-Animal Interaction Organizations 2018).

Animal-Assisted Interventions

The evidence surrounding the efficacy of AAIs for the treatment of depression is distributed across populations, purposes, and the developmental spectrum. For the purposes of our discussion, we provide a sampling of this literature. When an AAI is applied as a complementary therapy for the treatment of pain, it has been shown to significantly improve pain while also treating common mental health comorbidities including depression (Graham and Bair 2019). When trauma survivors and children and adults with symptoms of PTSD participated in an AAI, two systematic reviews indicated some evidence of reduced PTSD symptoms (Hediger et al. 2021) as well as reduced depression and anxiety (O'Haire et al. 2015), but the methodology used in the studies covered by these reviews lacked rigor, and the results were not universally consistent. A review of the existing randomized controlled trials conducted involving university students reported that AAIs can provide short-term benefits for anxiety and stress, but the limited evidence available from randomized controlled trials is inconclusive with regard to the potential effect of AAIs on depression (Parbery-Clark et al. 2021). A preponderance of the evidence found that depression was reduced and mood was elevated after an AAI in people with dementia who were living in nursing homes (Aarskog et al. 2019). Furthermore, use of an AAI involving dogs or robotic animals was considered to be a promising approach to reducing depression and improving mood and quality of life among this population. Pilot programs have examined the association between canine visitation and symptoms of depression and anxiety among women hospitalized for pregnancy complications. Findings suggested that therapy dog visitation was associated with reduced depressive and anxiety symptoms among this group after one 60-minute session (Lynch et al. 2014).

Ecosystem-Based Approaches

Some AAIs are subsumed under the larger umbrella of *ecotherapy*, a term that summarizes activities that connect individuals with nature (Chaudhury and Banerjee 2020). Approaches range from viewing nature scenes to immersion in the natural environment and have been associated with psychological and physiological indicators of stress reduction (Berto 2014) and improvements in mood and anxiety (Summers and Vivian 2018). *Care farming* represents a thorough integration of AAIs with the natural environment. Predominant mainly in Europe, care farming involves pairing groups of people with depression or other psychiatric illnesses with a local farmer who facilitates activities such as feeding, milking, and grooming animals, along with barn maintenance. Group discussions and cooperative tasks are embedded in the program. Randomized controlled studies examining depression outcomes have not found significant postprogram differences between care farming and control groups; however, self-reported depression symptoms did decrease during the intervention, while scores on self-efficacy and coping measures increased (Pedersen et al. 2015). Although the effect of such programs on depression remains unclear, these interventions may provide valuable motivation, behavioral activation, and interpersonal support for depressed individuals struggling with social isolation. These programs also may be more appealing to depressed patients compared with traditional therapies.

Animal-Assisted Therapy

Mechanistically, AAT may enhance patient response to CBT through a series of sequential effects: 1) increasing engagement with therapy (Fine 2015), 2) facilitating rapport between patient and therapist (Fine 2015), 3) reducing anxiety that may interfere with therapeutic learning (Jones et al. 2019), and 4) improving executive functioning (motivation, attention, and self-regulation) (Pendry et al. 2020). In addition, interactions with a therapy animal with whom a patient is bonded may be associated with changes in hormones such as dopamine, endorphins, and oxytocin (Odendaal 2000).

Feasibility and Acceptability of Animal-Assisted Therapies

AATs are generally well received among patients and staff with appropriate safety guidelines and preparation. In a study evaluating the effect of self-selected group AAT compared with group stress management therapy, both groups experienced reductions in depressive and anxiety symptoms, but the AAT group sessions were more well attended (Nepps et al. 2014).

Animal-Assisted Therapy in Specific Populations

Military veterans frequently return from service with depressive disorders secondary to psychological trauma or traumatic brain injury (TBI). Kinney et al. (2019) reviewed three studies (Ferruolo 2016; Lanning and Krenek 2013; Nevins et al. 2013) involving equine-assisted interventions or therapy targeting depressive symptoms in veterans with either comorbid PTSD or TBI. Program length ranged from 3 days to 6 months across studies and included a wide variety of activities such as body language and communication, groundwork (obstacle courses, stopping, backing up), and riding. Participants reported decreased depressive symptoms, increased perception of social support, and enhanced resilience following program participation. Hypothesized mechanisms for these effects were the unique experience of the horse-human bond, socialization with other people during the program, use of the horse as a "mirror" of one's own experience and behavior, mindfulness, development of autonomy, and the horse's natural calming effects on people.

Equine-facilitated psychotherapy may have unique effects on adolescent depression, anxiety, and behavior problems (Lentini and Knox 2015). Incorporating equines into treatment engages youth in ways that may break down barriers, which is characteristic of traditional "talk" therapy. Wilson et al. (2017) suggested that interacting with horses allows adolescents to build relationships with the animals more quickly than they would with humans and navigate the social discomfort of therapy more easily through active physical participation rather than passive conversation. Furthermore, working with horses allows young people to evaluate the effect of their behaviors by receiving immediate feedback from the animals.

Quality and Strength of Evidence for Animal-Assisted Interventions and Therapy in Depressed Populations

Generally speaking, evidence indicates a broad potential for AAIs to be used as a complementary depression treatment for a wide variety of populations in many settings. Short-term effects are found with relative consistency, but we do not fully understand the existence of, or potential for, long-term effects of AAIs. Furthermore, it is unclear whether a real dog is needed or if a robotic dog would be equally effective, or what specific aspects of the intervention are required to achieve the best benefit. With that said, there is good reason to consider AAIs as an adjunct to ongoing treatment of depression for those individuals who self-select for involvement with animals and who are unlikely to be aggressive toward animals. The evidence for AAIs is stronger than for pet ownership (described in the next section), and AAIs do not require the patient to be responsible for the animal's care or well-being.

Mounting evidence indicates that AAT is associated with improvement in depressive symptoms in specific populations. A range of small to large effect sizes (0.48–1.40) favoring AAT were reported in four studies of depression outcomes among adult psychiatric inpatients and those receiving nursing home care (Souter and Miller 2007). A meta-analysis of 9 clinical trials that included 447 participants produced a weighted pooled effect size of – 0.34, indicating a small effect size for reduction of depressive symptoms (Virues-Ortega et al. 2012). When only controlled trials were included in the analyses, the effect size increased to – 0.48, nearing the medium range. In a review of 18 controlled studies in health care settings that included dog-assisted interventions, activities, or therapy to address mental health outcomes, consistent improvements were reported for a variety of psychiatric outcome measures, including mood, emotional-behavioral symptoms, global functioning, and cortisol level (Lundqvist et al. 2017). In a review of 12 studies of depression outcomes among people with depression and/or anxiety disorders (5 randomized controlled trials and 7 involving dogs), 6 of the studies reported significant improvements in depressive symptoms (Eke and Mitchell 2019).

Although current evidence indicates that AAT can be effective in the treatment of depression, early reviews of existing randomized controlled trials found that studies were of relatively low quality (Kamioka et al. 2014) and did not provide sufficient scientific support for the use of AAT alone in the treatment of depression in adults (Charry-Sánchez et al. 2018). AAT may be more or less effective in different settings or at different points in time along the developmental spectrum. In hospitalized children and teenagers, especially those who have cancer, AAT was beneficial for controlling pain and blood pressure but did not make a significant difference in depression or anxiety (Feng et al. 2021). In adolescents, some evidence indicates that AAT may reduce depression symptoms in self-selected populations and improve subjective mood states (Jones et al. 2019).

Although evidence indicates that AAT is associated with improvement in depressive symptoms, as measured by self-report and standardized scales in specific populations, in those with severe dementia, the presence of the dog may not reduce symptoms but instead may act to reduce triggering or forestall the progression of some symptoms. Overall, the available evidence on AAT in the treatment of depression in older adults indicates that it is effective in reducing depression, but the evidence is not universally consistent (Charry-Sánchez et al. 2018).

Pet Ownership and Depression

A systematic review of literature published in 2017 found the evidence surrounding companion animal ownership to be inconclusive with regard to effects on childhood anxiety and depression (Purewal et al. 2017). Another, more recent review indicated that pet ownership may have nuanced effects on mental health (Scoresby et al. 2021). For example, women with pets tend to have lower levels of depression than do men with pets, and pet owners with severe mental illness had fewer hospitalizations than their non-pet-owning counterparts. However, older adults and single adults living alone who owned pets had higher levels of depression and loneliness than did those who did not own pets. Other studies replicated the relationship between sex, pet ownership, and depressive symptoms while providing conflicting results regarding the role of marital status. In one such study, the relationship between dog ownership and depression was moderated by both sex and marital status, with women and single dog owners reporting lower levels of depression than men and married individuals (Cline 2010). The relationship between pet ownership and depression is likely moderated by several individual characteristics, and further studies are needed to elucidate these relationships.

Study participants routinely indicate that their pets positively contribute to their mental health and well-being (Scoresby et al. 2021). Therefore, it is likely that depressed individuals may "self-treat" by acquiring a pet because they believe that the pet will positively contribute to their mental health. Research on pet ownership is predominantly correlational in nature, leaving us to discuss associations rather than causal relationships. If we find that pet owners have higher levels of depression, we do not know if those individuals were already depressed before acquiring the pet, and at the time of measurement, their depression levels may actually be reduced relative to their starting point. Likewise, when we find that pet owners have lower levels of depression, we do not ultimately know whether it was the pet who was responsible for reducing the depression or other potential variables (e.g., increased exercise, socialization).

Pet ownership research is murky for many reasons, not the least of which is that people like to select their own pets rather than having a researcher assign one to them. This self-selection bias leaves us asking the same question: does owning a pet improve health, or do healthier people opt to own pets? Finally, the ability to have and properly care for a pet requires a certain level of mental and physical health, combined with key resources, such as the ability to purchase food and provide housing for the animal. Together, these things suggest that over the long term, people who become hospitalized or homeless may struggle to continue to maintain their pet, effectively eliminating those individuals from the pet ownership category. Thus, pet owners may include a smaller proportion of frail, unhealthy, or impoverished individuals than non–pet owners. This idea is supported by a study that examined patterns of pet ownership among older adults (Friedmann et al. 2020). Pet ownership declines at older ages, an overall change that reflects the general pattern of reduced physical and mental health.

Companion Animals and Treatment-Resistant Depression

A significant proportion of people with MDD fail to respond to traditional, evidence-based treatments (Rush et al. 2006). Research efforts have typically focused on prescribing algorithms and treatment augmentation strategies to facilitate symptom relief (Voineskos et al. 2020). Some evidence suggests that adopting a dog or cat may be associated with depression response and remission for these patients. Mota Pereira and Fonte (2018) asked patients with treatment-resistant depression to self-select pet adoption or membership in a control group. Both groups received stable pharmacotherapy consistent with established prescribing guidelines for treatment-resistant depression. Significant improvements in depressive symptoms and global assessment of functioning were seen in the pet adoption group at 12 weeks postadoption compared with control subjects. The control group had no responders or remitters. Although attributions of causation are not possible given the lack of randomization in the study, this work represents an encouraging avenue for more rigorous, controlled studies of whether pet adoption plays a causal role in ameliorating intractable symptoms of depression. Such research should also explore animal welfare outcomes given that people with treatment-resistant depression are frequently hospitalized or experience difficulty completing self-care and other daily activities, which could affect the care a pet receives.

Clinical and Animal Welfare Considerations

Animals may play a significant role in facilitating recovery for people with depressive disorders. However, attention must be paid to the welfare and well-being of therapy animals and pets involved in helping people recover from depression. Many features of depressive disorders interfere with daily activities such as self-care, household management, employment, and socialization. Care must be taken to help patients thoroughly evaluate whether they have the personal and financial resources to care for a companion animal and to identify a surrogate caregiver for the animal in the event of psychiatric decompensation or hospitalization.

Additionally, symptoms of agitation, self-harm, and suicidality may distress therapy animals and pets, given animals' often keen awareness of human emotions. Sarlon et al. (2018) presented a case study of a wheaten terrier adopted by a woman with treatment-resistant depression and chronic suicidal ideation. Observations of the dog during his owner's psychiatric hospitalization suggested that the dog perceived the woman's distress and showed significant fear in response. When the woman experienced extreme agitation while discussing her plan for suicide during a crisis intervention session, the dog was seen cowering and shaking. The dog's behavior was attributed to the woman's crisis state given that the dog did not typically have these responses despite staying with his owner in an inpatient environment (Sarlon et al. 2018). Although global conclusions cannot be drawn from case studies, human-animal relationships are certainly bidirectional, making it important to study the effects of human psychiatric distress on therapy and companion animals and take steps to ensure their welfare and overall quality of life.

Case Example

Ms. L, a 45-year-old woman, had struggled with MDD since adolescence, as well as broken relationships, lost employment opportunities, and a pervasive sense of social isolation. Her illness was characterized by periods of great improvement and discouraging relapse. During extremely low points, Ms. L experienced painful episodes of hopelessness characterized by thoughts of ending her life. She was referred for crisis stabilization services during one particularly difficult episode. During an intake interview, the provider asked Ms. L to share her reasons for living—the considerations that made her question whether suicide was truly what she wanted when she experienced painful symptoms. Ms. L told the intake worker that she would never attempt suicide while her cat Milo was alive because she felt a sense of maternal responsibility for him and would not want to cause him pain or have anyone else take care of him. Milo was a powerful source of connection and responsibility for Ms. L that kept thoughts of suicide from evolving into attempts.

Ms. L's reasons for living provide a glimpse of the powerful attachment roles that companion animals can serve in the lives of people dealing with depressive disorders and other mental illnesses. Animals are often viewed as nonjudgmental and free from stigmatizing beliefs about people, making it feel safer for people to develop emotional connections with them. This case also highlights the need to help people with chronic mental illness plan for their companion animals in the event of symptom exacerbation and the need for inpatient or residential treatment.

Key Clinical Points

- Animal-assisted interventions (AAIs) and therapies (AATs) can augment evidence-based psychotherapeutic and pharmacological depression treatment but should not serve as a replacement for these approaches.

- Evidence suggests that AAIs and AATs may ameliorate depressive symptoms in the context of comorbidities such as chronic pain, PTSD, and dementia.

- Therapy animals may foster patients' engagement in treatment, particularly in the case of adolescents, who may be reluctant to participate in traditional "talk" therapy.

- Animals can provide immediate, nonjudgmental feedback regarding patients' behavior in more palatable ways than providers can.

- Interacting with animals may uniquely affect symptoms of anhedonia and low motivation.

- Adopting a companion animal may stimulate treatment response in those with treatment-resistant depressive disorder.

- Pet ownership is associated with reduced depressive symptoms for some individuals, with the effect being more robust in women and single people.

- Animal welfare must be considered when symptoms of agitation, suicidality, or self-injurious behavior predominate in a patient's clinical presentation.

- Treatment plans should account for companion animal welfare in the event of a patient's psychiatric decompensation or hospitalization.

References

Aarskog NK, Hunskår I, Bruvik F: Animal-assisted interventions with dogs and robotic animals for residents with dementia in nursing homes: a systematic review. Phys Occup Ther Geriatr 37(2):77–93, 2019

American Psychiatric Association: Diagnostic and Statistical Manual of Mental Disorders, 5th Edition, Text Revision. Washington, DC, American Psychiatric Association, 2022

American Psychological Association: Clinical Practice Guideline for the Treatment of Depression Across Three Age Cohorts. Washington, DC, American Psychological Association, 2019. Available at: https://www.apa.org/depression-guideline. Accessed January 29, 2022.

Berto R: The role of nature in coping with psycho-physiological stress: a literature review on restorativeness. Behav Sci (Basel) 4(4):394–409, 2014 25431444

Charry-Sánchez JD, Pradilla I, Talero-Gutiérrez C: Animal-assisted therapy in adults: a systematic review. Complement Ther Clin Pract 32:169–180, 2018 30057046

Chaudhury P, Banerjee D: "Recovering with nature": a review of ecotherapy and implications for the COVID-19 pandemic. Front Public Health 8:604440, 2020 33363096

Cline KM: Psychological effects of dog ownership: role strain, role enhancement, and depression. J Soc Psychol 150(2):117–131, 2010 20397589

Eke E, Mitchell CR: PMH1 animal assisted therapy (AAT) in depression and anxiety: a systematic review. Value Health 22(Suppl 3):S681, 2019

Feng Y, Lin Y, Zhang N, et al: Effects of animal-assisted therapy on hospitalized children and teenagers: a systematic review and meta-analysis. J Pediatr Nurs 60:11–23, 2021 33582447

Ferruolo DM: Psychosocial equine program for veterans. Soc Work 61(1):53–60, 2016 26897999

Fine AH: Incorporating animal-assisted interventions into psychotherapy: guidelines and suggestions for therapists, in Handbook on Animal-Assisted

Therapy, 4th Edition. Edited by Fine A. San Diego, CA, Elsevier, 2015, pp 141–155

Friedmann E, Gee NR, Simonsick EM, et al: Pet ownership patterns and successful aging outcomes in community dwelling older adults. Front Vet Sci 7:293, 2020 32671105

Giano Z, Ernst CW, Snider K, et al: ACE domains and depression: investigating which specific domains are associated with depression in adulthood. Child Abuse Negl 122:105335, 2021

Graham JD, Bair MJ: Animal assisted interventions to treat pain and associated mental health comorbidities: a systematized review. Proceedings of IMPRS 2(1), 2019

Harris EC, Barraclough B: Suicide as an outcome for mental disorders: a meta-analysis. Br J Psychiatry 170(3):205–228, 1997 9229027

Hasin DS, Sarvet AL, Meyers JL, et al: Epidemiology of adult DSM-5 major depressive disorder and its specifiers in the United States. JAMA Psychiatry 75(4):336–346, 2018 29450462

Hediger K, Wagner J, Künzi P, et al: Effectiveness of animal-assisted interventions for children and adults with post-traumatic stress disorder symptoms: a systematic review and meta-analysis. Eur J Psychotraumatol 12(1):1879713, 2021 34377357

International Association of Human-Animal Interaction Organizations: The IAHAIO Definitions for Animal Assisted Intervention and Guidelines for Wellness of Animals Involved in AAI. Seattle, WA, IAHAIO, 2018. Available at: https://iahaio.org/best-practice/white-paper-on-animal-assisted-interventions. Accessed April 16, 2018.

Jones MG, Rice SM, Cotton SM: Incorporating animal-assisted therapy in mental health treatments for adolescents: a systematic review of canine assisted psychotherapy. PLoS One 14(1):e0210761, 2019 30653587

Kamioka H, Okada S, Tsutani K, et al: Effectiveness of animal-assisted therapy: a systematic review of randomized controlled trials. Complement Ther Med 22(2):371–390, 2014 24731910

Katon WJ: Clinical and health services relationships between major depression, depressive symptoms, and general medical illness. Biol Psychiatry 54:216–226, 2003

Kessler RC, Bromet EJ: The epidemiology of depression across cultures. Annu Rev Public Health 34:119–138, 2013

Kessler RC, Foster CL, Saunders WB, Stang PE: Social consequences of psychiatric disorders, I: educational attainment. Am J Psychiatry 152(7):1026–1032, 1995 7793438

Kinney AR, Eakman AM, Lassell R, Wood W: Equine-assisted interventions for veterans with service-related health conditions: a systematic mapping review. Mil Med Res 6(1):28, 2019 31462305

Lanning BA, Krenek N: Guest editorial: examining effects of equine-assisted activities to help combat veterans improve quality of life. J Rehabil Res Dev 50(8):vii–xiii, 2013 24458903

Lentini JA, Knox MS: Equine-facilitated psychotherapy with children and adolescents: an update and literature review. J Creat Ment Health 10(3):278–305, 2015

Lundqvist M, Carlsson P, Sjödahl R, et al: Patient benefit of dog-assisted interventions in health care: a systematic review. BMC Complement Altern Med 17(1):358, 2017 28693538

Lynch CE, Magann EF, Barringer SN, et al: Pet therapy program for antepartum high-risk pregnancies: a pilot study. J Perinatol 34(11):816–818, 2014 24968176

Merikangas KR, Ames M, Cui L, et al: The impact of comorbidity of mental and physical conditions on role disability in the US adult household population. Arch Gen Psychiatry 64(10):1180–1188, 2007 17909130

Mojtabai R, Stuart EA, Hwang I, et al: Long-term effects of mental disorders on marital outcomes in the National Comorbidity Survey ten-year follow-up. Soc Psychiatry Psychiatr Epidemiol 52(10):1217–1226, 2017 28378065

Mota Pereira J, Fonte D: Pets enhance antidepressant pharmacotherapy effects in patients with treatment resistant major depressive disorder. J Psychiatr Res 104:108–113, 2018 30025233

Moussavi S, Chatterji S, Verdes E, et al: Depression, chronic diseases, and decrements in health: results from the World Health Surveys. Lancet 370(9590):851–858, 2007 17826170

Nepps P, Stewart CN, Bruckno SR: Animal-assisted activity: effects of a complementary intervention program on psychological and physiological variables. J Evid Based Complementary Altern Med 19(3):211–215, 2014 24789913

Nevins R, Finch S, Hickling EJ, Barnett SD: The Saratoga WarHorse project: a case study of the treatment of psychological distress in a veteran of Operation Iraqi Freedom. Adv Mind Body Med 27(4):22–25, 2013 24067322

Nock MK, Hwang I, Sampson N, et al: Cross-national analysis of the associations among mental disorders and suicidal behavior: findings from the WHO World Mental Health Surveys. PLoS Med 6(8):e1000123, 2009 19668361

Odendaal JS: Animal-assisted therapy: magic or medicine? J Psychosom Res 49(4):275–280, 2000 11119784

O'Haire ME, Guérin NA, Kirkham AC: Animal-assisted intervention for trauma: a systematic literature review. Front Psychol 6:1121, 2015 26300817

Parbery-Clark C, Lubamba M, Tanner L, McColl E: Animal-assisted interventions for the improvement of mental health outcomes in higher education students: a systematic review of randomised controlled trials. Int J Environ Res Public Health 18(20):10768, 2021 34682513

Pedersen I, Patil G, Berget B, et al: Mental health rehabilitation in a care farm context: a descriptive review of Norwegian intervention studies. Work 53(1):31–43, 2015 26684702

Pendry P, Carr AM, Gee NR, Vandagriff JL: Randomized trial examining effects of animal assisted intervention and stress related symptoms on college students' learning and study skills. Int J Environ Res Public Health 17(6):1909–1926, 2020 32183453

Purewal R, Christley R, Kordas K, et al: Companion animals and child/adolescent development: a systematic review of the evidence. Int J Environ Res Public Health 14(3):234, 2017 28264460

Rohde P, Beevers CG, Stice E, O'Neil K: Major and minor depression in female adolescents: onset, course, symptom presentation, and demographic associations. J Clin Psychol 65(12):1339–1349, 2009 19827116

Rush AJ, Trivedi MH, Wisniewski SR, et al: Acute and longer-term outcomes in depressed outpatients requiring one or several treatment steps: a STAR*D report. Am J Psychiatry 163(11):1905–1917, 2006 17074942

Sarlon J, Staniloiu A, Schöntges A, Kordon A: Vegetative symptoms and behaviour of the therapy-accompanying dog of a chronically suicidal patient. BMJ Case Rep 2018:bcr2018225483, 2018 30150341

Scoresby KJ, Strand EB, Ng Z, et al: Pet ownership and quality of life: a systematic review of the literature. Vet Sci 8(12):332, 2021 34941859

Souter MA, Miller MD: Do animal-assisted activities effectively treat depression? A meta-analysis. Anthrozoos 20(2):167–180, 2007

Summers JK, Vivian DN: Ecotherapy: a forgotten ecosystem service. A review. Front Psychol 9:1389, 2018 30123175

Virues-Ortega J, Pastor-Barriuso R, Castellote JM, Poblacion A: Effect of animal-assisted therapy on the psychological and functional status of elderly populations and patients with psychiatric disorders: a meta-analysis. Health Psychol Rev 6(2):197–221, 2012

Voineskos D, Daskalakis ZJ, Blumberger DM: Management of treatment-resistant depression: challenges and strategies. Neuropsychiatr Dis Treat 16:221–234, 2020 32021216

Wang PS, Simon G, Kessler RC: The economic burden of depression and the cost-effectiveness of treatment. Int J Methods Psychiatr Res 12(1):22–33, 2003 12830307

Wilson K, Buultjens M, Monfries M, Karimi L: Equine-assisted psychotherapy for adolescents experiencing depression and/or anxiety: a therapist's perspective. Clin Child Psychol Psychiatry 22(1):16–33, 2017 26668260

Wisner KL, Sit DKY, McShea MC, et al: Onset timing, thoughts of self-harm, and diagnoses in postpartum women with screen-positive depression findings. JAMA Psychiatry 70(5):490–498, 2013

9

Companion Animals in the Treatment of Stress and Anxiety

Erika Friedmann, Ph.D.
Nancy R. Gee, Ph.D.
James Levenson, M.D.

WE BRIEFLY DESCRIBE psychological stress and anxiety disorders, explain the physiological changes occurring during stress and anxiety, and then review the relevant human-animal interaction (HAI) research suggestive of possible roles for companion animals in moderating these physiological stress responses. We discuss evidence that HAI affects stress and anxiety, and we review research addressing the incorporation of HAI into mental health treatment and the use of HAI as a complementary and adjunctive therapy to reduce anxiety in psychiatric patients with other diagnoses. Finally, we describe the potential uses of HAI for stress and anxiety disorders. PTSD is discussed separately in Chapter 10 ("Companion Animals in the Treatment of PTSD"). We conclude with specific examples and resources to aid the clinician in practical applications. We point the reader to Chapter 2 ("A Working Partnership

Between Clinicians and Therapy Dogs in the Treatment of Mental Disorders") to better understand the animal side of the equation and to Chapter 3 ("Roles of Animals With Individuals Who Have Mental Illness") for a fuller outline of the various roles of companion animals as well as the clinician's responsibilities in HAI.

Prevalence of Stress and Anxiety and Risk Factors

During the coronavirus SARS-CoV-2 disease (COVID-19) pandemic, the prevalence of stress and anxiety in the general population was estimated to be 29.6% and 31.9%, respectively (Salari et al. 2020). An estimated 19.1% of U.S. adults had any anxiety disorder in the past year, and about 31% of U.S. adults experience any anxiety disorder at some time in their lives (National Institute of Mental Health 2021); however, estimates of the prevalence of stress disorders have been largely limited to PTSD, with an estimated lifetime prevalence of PTSD by DSM-5 criteria (American Psychiatric Association 2022) of 8.3% in 2010 in the U.S. general population (Kilpatrick et al. 2013).

Risk factors for anxiety disorders include temperamental (e.g., neuroticism), environmental (e.g., adverse childhood experiences), genetic, and physiological (e.g., certain medications or substances) factors.

Clinical Presentation and Longitudinal Time Course

Psychological Stress

Stress is an experience of cognitive and emotional strain or pressure (Rom and Reznick 2015). It can result from environmental (e.g., workplace), interpersonal (e.g., marital conflict), or internal (e.g., unrealistic self-imposed demands) stimuli. Like anxiety, stress that is in proportion to circumstances is normal and unavoidable and may be beneficial. Stress activates psychological, behavioral, and physiological responses that assist individuals in confronting or adapting to threats to their welfare. Too much stress is emotionally, cognitively, and physiologically harmful. Prolonged stress is associated with increased risk for myocardial infarction, cardiac arrhythmia, stroke, hypertension, peptic ulcer disease, and depression and can aggravate preexisting conditions, such as diabetes mellitus, epilepsy, and anxiety disorders.

Anxiety Disorders

Anxiety disorders are characterized by the experience of excessive anxiety and/or fear and related physiological and behavioral manifestations (Craske et al. 2017). Acute anxiety may be experienced in response to a real or perceived imminent threat, whereas sustained anxiety may be more focused on future danger. Various anxiety disorders differ in degree of hypervigilance, muscle tension, autonomic arousal, and avoidant behaviors (i.e., avoiding the feared situation), as well as thought processes and content. Anxiety encompasses a spectrum from normal to pathological. It reaches the level of a disorder when it is persistent (not just transient) and results in significant emotional distress and/or social or occupational impairment. When the feared situation is real, the distress and impairment are clearly disproportionate to how others would react to that situation. Anxiety as a symptom occurs in many other psychiatric disorders, and anxiety disorders frequently co-occur. Therefore, the most common anxiety disorder is not one of the specific types, but instead a combination that includes characteristics of two or more specific anxiety disorders. Anxiety disorders are frequently comorbid with substance use disorders and mood disorders, including depression (discussed in Chapter 8, "Companion Animals in the Treatment of Depressive Disorders"). In general, anxiety disorders begin in childhood or young adulthood and are more common in females than in males.

The most common anxiety disorder is generalized anxiety disorder, characterized by excessive anxiety and worrying most of the time (DeMartini et al. 2019). Sleep difficulties, fatigue, poor concentration, irritability, restlessness, and muscle tension are common manifestations. Treatment options include cognitive-behavioral therapy (CBT) and pharmacotherapy (most antidepressants).

Panic disorder is characterized by recurrent panic attacks, which are states of high autonomic arousal (Asmundson et al. 2014). Affected individuals may experience palpitations, diaphoresis, tremor, shortness of breath, chest tightness, nausea or other gastrointestinal distress, lightheadedness, paresthesia, and numbness. Also commonly experienced are an acute sense of impending doom and fear of losing control. Frequent uncontrolled panic attacks result in anticipatory anxiety (worrying about another panic attack) and avoidance of places or situations where a previous anxiety attack occurred, resulting in agoraphobia.

Agoraphobia is the fear of being out in a public place, especially if it is crowded or the person would be going alone (Asmundson et al. 2014). When the fear is severe, it may result in a person not leaving home at all.

Most but not all cases are associated with panic disorder. Treatment options include CBT and pharmacotherapy (antidepressants for maintenance treatment, benzodiazepines for acute attacks).

Social anxiety disorder is characterized by marked anxiety regarding situations in which the person fears how others will see or judge them, resulting in humiliation or embarrassment (Leichsenring and Leweke 2017). Typical feared situations include meeting new people at a party or reception or giving a presentation at work or in class. Social anxiety disorder was sometimes called *social phobia* and should not be conflated with normal shyness. First-line treatment is CBT, but antidepressants can be helpful in treatment. β-Blockers or benzodiazepines are sometimes prescribed before specific situations such as a presentation.

Specific (sometimes called *simple*) phobia is characterized by marked anxiety regarding a specific situation or thing (Eaton et al. 2018). Common animal phobias include fear of spiders, snakes, wasps, mice or rats, and dogs. Common health-related phobias include fear of needles/injections, blood, general anesthesia, and dentists. Other common phobias are fear of heights (acrophobia), flying, and enclosed spaces (claustrophobia). Behavioral therapy (desensitization, exposure) is the treatment of choice.

Physiological Underpinnings of Stress and Anxiety

Both stress and anxiety involve activation of the hypothalamic-pituitary-adrenal (HPA) axis and the sympathetic-adrenal-medulla (SAM) system (Musselman et al. 1998; Rozanski et al. 1999). SAM hyperactivity results in increased catecholamine release, reduced heart rate variability, and increased sympathetic tone. Activation of the HPA axis initiates a series of neurohormonal responses and releases corticosteroids into the bloodstream (Friedmann 2019). Activation of both systems causes several physiological changes; commonly used indicators of the degree of stress include increased blood pressure, heart rate, cortisol, cortisol awakening response, and α-amylase as well as decreased peripheral blood flow (peripheral skin temperature), heart rate variability, and immunoglobulins (Vogel et al. 2019). Scales commonly used to assess individuals' perceptions of their stress and anxiety levels include the Perceived Stress Scale (Lee 2012; Roberti et al. 2006), Spielberger's State-Trait Anxiety Inventory (Kabacoff et al. 1997), and the Beck Anxiety Inventory (Kabacoff et al. 1997). In research, these tools measure changes in symptoms (response and remission), not diagnoses.

Overview of Existing Evidence-Based Treatments

Evidence-based treatments for anxiety disorders include both pharmacotherapy and psychotherapy. CBT has the most empirical support among the psychotherapies. Cognitive and behavioral techniques used include psychoeducation, cognitive restructuring, in vivo exposure, self-monitoring, breathing retraining, muscle relaxation, and relapse prevention. There is also some evidence for the benefits of psychodynamic and interpersonal psychotherapies. The first-line pharmacological choice for most anxiety disorders is a selective serotonin reuptake inhibitor. Other options include serotonin-norepinephrine reuptake inhibitors, buspirone, and benzodiazepines. In treatment-resistant cases, a combination of more than one of the above, antipsychotics, and gabapentin may be considered. Benzodiazepines should be avoided in patients with a history of substance use disorders and those otherwise at increased risk for dependency or misuse. β-Blockers are the drug of choice for stage fright or other performance anxiety, but short-acting benzodiazepines are sometimes prescribed for this. For most anxiety disorders, the choice between psychotherapy and pharmacotherapy is based on patient preference, but the combination of both is more effective (Craske et al. 2017).

Potential for Companion Animals to Reduce Stress and Anxiety

The involvement of animals in the reduction of distress and the improvement of mental health predates the modern medical model and contemporary psychotherapy (Crossman 2017). The belief that animals improve human mental health dates back to the seventeenth century and is popularly endorsed today. Psychological distress is the most common mental health concern targeted by HAI-based interventions, known collectively as *animal-assisted interventions* (AAIs). An *animal-assisted activity* (AAA) is a form of AAI that typically provides humans the opportunity to interact with animals in an unscripted, or semistructured, way with the broad goal of improving mood and reducing perceived stress, physiological arousal, and anxiety. *Animal-assisted therapy* (AAT) is goal-directed and involves a health practitioner incorporating a trained animal into the treatment regimen for a specific disorder. Very little research has evaluated the efficacy of AAT in treating stress or anxiety.

According to Crossman (2017), HAI programs can be readily accessible, efficient, cost-effective, and appealing and widely scalable, but they are not intended to replace traditional psychotherapy or psychiatric medications. Rather, HAI programs may reduce or circumvent barriers to treatment and serve as an adjunct to traditional approaches. HAI programs tend to reduce stigma associated with traditional treatments and improve attendance and participation in treatment. People perceive AAI programs as credible and effective for improving mental health.

Scientific Evidence Base

Animals as Adjuncts in the Treatment of Anxiety in Psychiatric Patients

Although only a few studies have examined animals as adjuncts in the treatment of psychiatric patients, those studies suggested that AAAs are at least as effective at reducing anxiety during sessions as other therapeutic activities. Long-term improvements in anxiety over several sessions have not been investigated, and careless terminology resulted in some studies reporting the use of AAT, when AAA or AAI would have been more accurate. As is discussed in Chapter 3, AAT involves a licensed mental health professional incorporating an animal into a goal-directed therapeutic process, whereas an AAA is an activity involving an animal that is not goal-directed, and an AAI is a purposeful intervention that is goal-directed but does not necessarily involve a mental health professional.

Acute-care psychiatric inpatients who participated in 1-hour AAA or stress management sessions experienced similar significant reductions in anxiety, depression, and heart rate with the two interventions. Animal sessions were more popular than stress reduction sessions, and this indicated acceptability to the inpatients diagnosed with serious mental illnesses, including major depressive disorder, bipolar disorder, and schizophrenia (Nepps et al. 2014). In a crossover study comparing AAIs and therapeutic recreation, patients with psychotic disorders, mood disorders, and other disorders experienced reduced anxiety after the AAI; only patients with mood disorders experienced reduced anxiety after therapeutic recreation (Barker and Dawson 1998). In a much smaller study of 12 patients hospitalized with major depressive disorder, anxiety was lower after an AAA than after a control condition (Hoffmann et al. 2009). However, a crossover study comparing waiting with a dog and waiting with magazines before electroconvulsive therapy did not find differences in anxiety (Barker et al. 2003).

Although few studies have directly addressed the use of AAAs to reduce anxiety, a larger literature addresses one anxiety-related disorder, PTSD, and is discussed in Chapter 10.

Pet Ownership

Indirect evidence suggests that pet ownership may affect stress through its association with reduced stress-related disease mortality or total mortality (Friedmann 2019; Friedmann and Thomas 1995; Friedmann et al. 1980, 2011). However, limited attention has been paid to direct effects on stress. Some epidemiological studies describe differences in stress indicators between pet owners and those who do not own pets, with inconsistent results including lower (Anderson et al. 1992) and higher (Parslow and Jorm 2003) physiological stress indicators. A few studies of companion animals in a home setting suggested that the animal's presence reduced stress indicators, such as with the introduction of dogs into homes with autistic children (Viau et al. 2010). Of course, people choose their pets based on their attitudes, making it difficult to separate contributions of pet ownership and pet attitudes to any stress moderation experienced by pet owners (Serpell 1981).

Settings and Populations

On the basis of the evidence presented above, there is reason to argue that pet owners derive some stress and anxiety reductions from their own pets. There is also reason to believe that pets may *increase* stress and anxiety in their owners in some situations. Dogs with behavior problems may be challenging to walk on a leash or take to the veterinarian, groomer, or boarding kennel, making routine dog care stressful. In a study of 164 pet owners obtaining veterinary oncology services, caregiver burden was correlated with owners' higher stress, symptoms of depression, and lower quality of life (Shaevitz et al. 2020). In a qualitative study, older adults reported three sources of stress and anxiety as reasons for no longer owning pets: competing demands on time, burden of caregiving, and concern about the impending grieving process (Chur-Hansen et al. 2008).

An *emotional support animal* (ESA) is any species of animal that helps an individual cope with symptoms of a mental disability through their daily presence. Information about the role and involvement of

ESAs is addressed in Chapter 3. Little research addresses the efficacy of ESAs in improving health outcomes. In a small longitudinal pilot study, self-report measures of anxiety, depression, and loneliness decreased from before to after ESA acquisition (Hoy-Gerlach et al. 2021). However, physiological stress indicators did not change from before to 12 months after ESA acquisition.

Proximity Effects

Many studies of the effect of animals on human physiological stress indicators use experimental techniques to evaluate physiological responses to viewing or being in the presence of an animal. This research evaluates the effects of the animal on stress and on stress response buffering. Studies found that interacting with a friendly animal, not necessarily one's own pet, leads to direct antiarousal effects but not inevitably to stress response–moderating effects (Baun et al. 1984; Katcher 1981).

Direct and Moderating Stress Effects of Viewing Animals

Differences in physiological indicators of stress and subjective perceptions of stress as related to viewing an animal are not always correlated. For instance, in a study where university students observed aquariums both with and without fish, the students felt significantly more relaxed in the with-fish condition, but physiological indicators did not reflect lower stress (Gee et al. 2019). In contrast, in another aquarium observation study (Katcher et al. 1983), blood pressure increases in response to reading aloud were less pronounced after watching fish than after watching other stimuli.

Direct and Moderating Stress Effects of Being in the Presence of an Animal

One study found that being in the presence of animals affected indicators of physiological arousal and moderated children's stress responses (Friedmann et al. 1983). Evidence from PET scans showed that pet owners had less activity in brain regions associated with sympathetic nervous system arousal when their dogs were present during the scans than when they were not (Sugawara et al. 2012). A guinea pig's presence was effective at reducing social stress for children on the autism spectrum (O'Haire et al. 2015).

The presence of an unfamiliar, novel dog also resulted in decreased cortisol levels and reduced cardiovascular responses in college students throughout a series of tasks testing stress and anxiety (Polheber and Matchock 2014). A dog's presence reduced cardiovascular responses to the social stressor of reading aloud in front of others, as seen in children, college students, and community-living older adults (Baun et al. 1984; Katcher 1981). Note that a few studies found no reduction in stress responses in the presence of dogs (Rajack 1997).

The presence of animals also reduced stress in outpatient and inpatient health care settings. The presence of a friendly animal moderated young children's physiological stress responses in a simulated physical examination (Nagengast et al. 1997) and behavioral distress during outpatient visits (Hansen et al. 1999). Oncology patients who chose to have chemotherapy in a room with dogs present experienced less physiological stress than did those without dogs present (Orlandi et al. 2007). Similarly, physiological stress indicators were reduced for cardiac inpatients awaiting heart transplants who were exposed to a fish aquarium (Cole and Gawlinski 2000).

Possible Explanations for Stress Responses

As can be seen from the research just summarized, the presence of an animal moderates stress responses, but not uniformly. Positive perceptions of dogs promote dogs' effectiveness at reducing people's stress responses (Friedmann et al. 1993). College students with more positive attitudes toward dogs had lower cardiovascular stress responses to reading aloud in the presence of a dog than did those with less positive attitudes toward dogs (Friedmann et al. 1993). The presence of an animal may be beneficial only for individuals who are comfortable with the animals (Friedmann 2019).

The nonjudgmental aspect of the support from the animal is suggested as the basis for decreases in stress and anxiety when an animal is present. This is consistent with research indicating greater stress responses in the presence of more judgmental or authoritative individuals (Long et al. 1982).

Therapeutic Interactions With Animals

Nature of Interaction With Animal

A key question is whether physical contact with an animal is necessary or advantageous for reductions in stress or anxiety. It appears that the situation and the type of contact may play a role in determining what is most efficacious for reducing stress and anxiety (Friedmann 2019). In one study (Gee et al. 2014), touching a dog had no effect on autonomic arousal, and in another study, physiological arousal decreased the most without physical contact with the animal (Demello 1999). As noted later in this chapter, under other circumstances, touching animals has been found to have beneficial effects.

Settings and Populations

A survey of mental health professionals who use AAT in their practices indicated that most of them use five techniques: reflect or comment on the client's relationship with the therapy animal, encourage clients to interact with the animal by touching or petting them, comment or reflect on spontaneous client-animal interactions, have the therapy animal present without any directive interventions, and allow the therapy animal to engage with the client in spontaneous moments that facilitate therapeutic discussion. Most clinicians also share information about the dog's history and stories and metaphors about animals (O'Callaghan and Chandler 2011). We are unaware of any studies cataloging how patients/clients interact with dogs or other animals in therapeutic settings.

Therapy dog team visits that generally allow touching and talking to the dog have become popular for reducing stress on college campuses. Single sessions with therapy dogs last from approximately 15 minutes to more than 30 minutes. Data from studies of these programs provide evidence that the therapy dog visits reduce students' psychological stress (Barker et al. 2016; Binfet 2017; Ward-Griffin et al. 2018), physiological stress indicators (Krause-Parello 2012; Pendry and Vandagriff 2019), and anxiety (Grajfoner et al. 2017; Ward-Griffin et al. 2018). In studies of children (Beetz et al. 2011) and college students (Pendry and Vandagriff 2019), AAAs were more effective at reducing physiological stress indicators when participants touched the dogs than when they did not.

Health care professionals who interacted with a therapy dog for 5 minutes experienced decreased physiological stress indicators equivalent to those following 20 minutes of rest (Barker et al. 2005). Medical students and residents who interacted with a dog experienced greater reductions in anxiety than did comparable individuals who did not interact (Crossman et al. 2015). By contrast, adolescents showed no evidence that a canine AAA session with or without touch reduced physiological stress responses or anxiety (Mueller et al. 2021).

Hospitalized patients also experienced reduced physiological stress indicators or perceptions of stress in response to canine AAAs. Heart failure inpatients had significantly greater reductions in physiological stress indicators during and after an AAA compared with those receiving a visit from a human volunteer or usual care (Cole et al. 2007). Hospitalized acute-care patients experienced decreased perceptions of anxiety, as well as decreased cardiovascular stress indicators, after an AAA visit, but no comparison with a control condition was reported (Coakley et al. 2021).

Hospitalized children had greater reductions in physiological stress indicators (Tsai et al. 2010) and anxiety (Barker et al. 2015) with AAT than with another child life intervention, and interacting with a dog reduced anxiety in children preparing to undergo MRI (Perez et al. 2019). By contrast, physiological stress indicators of children awakening from anesthesia did not differ based on the presence of a dog (Calcaterra et al. 2015).

Research shows that the presence of an animal is associated with both reduced stress and anxiety and reduced stress and anxiety responses to stressors in at least some populations or situations. The usefulness of AAAs or AAIs for reducing stress or distress likely depends on patients' initial conditions; individuals with more stress seemed to derive more benefit (Havener et al. 2001). This suggests the relevance of examining the use of AAAs and AAIs for reducing stress and anxiety in patients with anxiety-related disorders.

Quality and Strength of Evidence Base and Limitations

It can be difficult to assess stress and anxiety reduction stemming from pet ownership because pet ownership is seldom assigned to participants in a study. When pet ownership is not randomly assigned, we cannot determine whether healthier people opt to own pets or whether pets may help people to be healthier. Furthermore, it is nearly impossible to blind participants and study personnel to the presence of the animal, which may influence results.

The results of AAI studies are more solidly based, if not always consistent. As with most research into HAI, recent years have seen improvements in study design, but unfortunately very few of these studies include a longitudinal evaluation. In emerging treatment areas such as ESAs, there is a paucity of research, and professionals must rely almost exclusively on anecdotal, self-report, and qualitative evidence. Several large-scale randomized clinical trials are needed to seriously entertain prescribing pets to help people cope with their mental illnesses.

A common caveat in studies of HAI is that they include only people who expressed an interest in participating in studies with the animals. However, anecdotal evidence suggests that people may change their views of animals on the basis of their experiences. If animals are introduced in a positive way, patients or others who were initially fearful may become less so or even look forward to their presence with repeated exposures.

Implications for Clinical Practice

Research suggests that having an animal present could be beneficial in reducing stress and anxiety during therapeutic encounters or in the homes of individuals with anxiety-related disorders. Studies of stress-moderating effects of interacting with animals suggest that the situation might determine the clinical benefit of HAI. Under some circumstances, the presence of a dog or the way the interactions are structured may actually increase stress and anxiety rather than act as a therapeutic agent. This places the responsibility for evaluating the patient and the situation, and the appropriateness of including animals as adjunctive modalities in the therapeutic milieu, on the practitioner.

It is important for clinicians to remember that although companion animals may provide a way to reach, connect with, and treat many patients, they are not a panacea. Not all patients respond to, or even like, companion animals. Best practice is to communicate openly and directly with patients about whether they would like an animal included in their treatment plans. Not all patients will treat animals humanely or with respect and kindness or be capable of providing appropriate care. It is important to limit inclusion of animals in treatment to those individuals who will act humanely with them. Actively monitoring patients' behavior and interaction during activities with animals is crucial for the safety of both the patients and the animals. The practitioner must be prepared to safely remove the animal if warranted. Chapters 2 and 3 include more information about animal welfare considerations and clinicians' responsibilities while including animals in therapeutic settings.

Tables 9–1, 9–2, and 9–3 provide example skills for use with patients who own pets (column 1), patients who may interact with therapy dog/handler teams in an AAA setting (column 2), and mental health practitioners who incorporate AAT into their therapeutic practices (column 3).

Table 9–1. Example skill #1: relaxation—mindfulness

At home with pet dog	Animal-assisted activity	Animal-assisted therapy
Suggest that patients sit with their dog while the dog is relaxed and sleeping and gently stroke their dog and • Match their breathing to their dog's. • Sense the dog's body as they stroke the dog. Is it warm? Is it soft? • Imagine what the animal may be dreaming about.	Invite a therapy dog/handler team to interact freely with patients while they wait in a waiting room. • Invite the handler to walk slowly around the room, letting people pet the dog. • Ask the handler to focus the conversation on all the relaxing things the dog enjoys, such as where the dog likes to be stroked. • Give the dog a bone to chew and observe their enjoyment.	During a therapeutic session, lead a mindfulness exercise focused on a sleeping dog. • Watch the dog's chest rise and fall. • Listen to the dog's breathing. Imagine what it feels like to touch the dog. • Can you feel the warmth of the dog's body?

Table 9–2. Example skill #2: stress reduction—physical activity

At home with pet dog	Animal-assisted activity	Animal-assisted therapy
Suggest that patients consider doing distracting interactive activities with their dogs: doga, dog fitness, obedience, agility, rally, tricks, flyball, or others. For descriptions of these activities and more ideas, visit www.akc.org.	Incorporate therapy dog movement-based activities into the patient's overall treatment plan. Activities can include walking the dog with a dual leash, playing fetch, working with the dog to perform tricks, and grooming the dog.	During a therapeutic session, if a patient becomes dysregulated and in need of an activity to calm and refocus them, consider stopping the session and going for a walk with the dog. Allow the patient time to reflect and focus and return to the session when ready.

Table 9–3.   Example skill #3: treatment goal: anxiety reduction and management

At home with pet dog	Animal-assisted activity	Animal-assisted therapy
Describe a tool such as mindfulness as a way to replace a specific maladaptive behavior or thought pattern.		
Suggest that patients take their dog for a walk and focus on mindfulness throughout the walk.	Invite a therapy dog/handler team to interact freely with patients while they wait in a waiting room.	Demonstrate mindfully watching a resting dog.
• What is the dog interested in?	• Invite the handler to walk slowly around the room, letting people pet the dog.	• Focus on the resting dog's breathing and try to match your breathing rate to that of the dog.
• Where does the dog want to go?	• Ask the handler to focus the conversation on all the relaxing things the dog enjoys such as where the dog likes to be stroked.	• Focus completely on the dog and all aspects of the resting dog.
• What does the weather of the day feel like? Is it cold, hot, humid, overcast?	• Give the dog a toy to play with and observe their focus on, and enjoyment of, the toy.	• Describe how it feels to stroke the dog, and discuss what the dog might be dreaming about.
• Can you smell anything like fresh-cut grass, or food cooking, or nearby flowers?		
• What does the grass, pavement, or ground feel like beneath your feet?		

Resources

The following set of resources might be useful for implementing AAT in practice.

Continuing education, standards of practice, competencies, and accreditations	Animal Assisted Intervention International	https://aai-int.org
Certification: animal-assisted intervention specialist	Pet Partners/ Association of Animal-Assisted Intervention Professionals	https://petpartners.org/ learn/aat-professionals
Certificate as a human-animal intervention specialist	Center for Human Animal Interventions, Oakland University	https://oakland.edu/ nursing/continuing-education/ animalassistedtherapy
Human-animal studies courses	Animals & Society Institute	https://www. animalsandsociety.org/ resources/resources-for-students/degree-programs

Key Clinical Points

- Animal-assisted interventions (AAIs)—both animal-assisted activities (AAAs) and animal-assisted therapy (AAT)—may help circumvent barriers to treatment for individuals with anxiety or depression as an adjunct to traditional clinical or pharmacological treatments. They are not considered a stand-alone option.

- Research suggests that AAIs may be most effective in reducing stress when the initial stress level is high, although more research is necessary to confirm this indication.

- The nature of an effective intervention will depend on the circumstances of each patient. For instance, touching an animal during an intervention may have a therapeutic effect, although for some patients and treatment modalities, being in the presence of the animal may be sufficient.

- Patients should be consulted in advance about their comfort level regarding including an animal in a therapeutic treatment plan.

- Clinicians must be responsible for assessing patient responses to AAIs and for moderating or terminating interactions in which stress or anxiety may actually increase in the presence of an animal.

- Animal welfare must be an important consideration in any AAI. If a patient does not treat an animal humanely during an intervention, the animal should be removed immediately.

References

American Psychiatric Association: Diagnostic and Statistical Manual of Mental Disorders, 5th Edition, Text Revision. Washington, DC, American Psychiatric Association, 2022

Anderson WP, Reid CM, Jennings GL: Pet ownership and risk factors for cardiovascular disease. Med J Aust 157(5):298–301, 1992 1435469

Asmundson GJ, Taylor S, Smits JA: Panic disorder and agoraphobia: an overview and commentary on DSM-5 changes. Depress Anxiety 31(6):480–486, 2014 24865357

Barker SB, Dawson KS: The effects of animal-assisted therapy on anxiety ratings of hospitalized psychiatric patients. Psychiatr Serv 49(6):797–801, 1998 9634160

Barker SB, Pandurangi AK, Best AM: Effects of animal-assisted therapy on patients' anxiety, fear, and depression before ECT. J ECT 19(1):38–44, 2003 12621276

Barker SB, Knisely JS, McCain NL, Best AM: Measuring stress and immune response in healthcare professionals following interaction with a therapy dog: a pilot study. Psychol Rep 96(3 Pt 1):713–729, 2005 16050629

Barker SB, Knisely JS, Schubert CM, et al: The effect of an animal-assisted intervention on anxiety and pain in hospitalized children. Anthrozoos 28(1):101–112, 2015

Barker SB, Barker RT, McCain NL, Schubert CM: A randomized cross-over exploratory study of the effect of visiting therapy dogs on college student stress before final exams. Anthrozoos 29(1):35–46, 2016

Baun MM, Bergstrom N, Langston NF, Thoma L: Physiological effects of human/companion animal bonding. Nurs Res 33(3):126–129, 1984 6563527

Beetz A, Kotrschal K, Turner DC, et al: The effect of a real dog, toy dog and friendly person on insecurely attached children during a stressful task: an exploratory study. Anthrozoos 24(4):349–368, 2011

Binfet JT: The effects of group-administered canine therapy on university students' wellbeing: a randomized controlled trial. Anthrozoos 30(3):397–414, 2017

Calcaterra V, Veggiotti P, Palestrini C, et al: Post-operative benefits of animal-assisted therapy in pediatric surgery: a randomised study. PLoS One 10(6):e0125813, 2015 26039494

Chur-Hansen A, Winefield H, Beckwith M: Reasons given by elderly men and women for not owning a pet, and the implications for clinical practice and research. J Health Psychol 13(8):988–995, 2008 18987070

Coakley AB, Annese CD, Empoliti JH, Flanagan JM: The experience of animal assisted therapy on patients in an acute care setting. Clin Nurs Res 30(4):401–405, 2021 33242977

Cole KM, Gawlinski A: Animal-assisted therapy: the human-animal bond. AACN Clin Issues 11(1):139–149, 2000 11040560

Cole KM, Gawlinski A, Steers N, Kotlerman J: Animal-assisted therapy in patients hospitalized with heart failure. Am J Crit Care 16(6):575–585, quiz 586, discussion 587–588, 2007 17962502

Craske MG, Stein MB, Eley TC, et al: Correction: anxiety disorders. Nat Rev Dis Primers 3:17100, 2017

Crossman MK: Effects of interactions with animals on human psychological distress. J Clin Psychol 73(7):761–784, 2017 27809353

Crossman MK, Kazdin AE, Knudson K: Brief unstructured interaction with a dog reduces distress. Anthrozoos 28(4):649–659, 2015

DeMartini J, Patel G, Fancher TL: Generalized anxiety disorder. Ann Intern Med 170(7):ITC49–ITC64, 2019 30934083

Demello LR: The effect of the presence of a companion-animal on physiological changes following the termination of cognitive stressors. Psychol Health 14(5):859–868, 1999

Eaton WW, Bienvenu OJ, Miloyan B: Specific phobias. Lancet Psychiatry 5(8):678–686, 2018 30060873

Friedmann E: The animal-human bond: health and wellness, in Handbook on Animal-Assisted Therapy: Foundations and Guidelines for Animal-Assisted Interventions, 5th Edition. Edited by Fine AH. London, Academic Press, 2019, pp 79–100

Friedmann E, Thomas SA: Pet ownership, social support, and one-year survival after acute myocardial infarction in the Cardiac Arrhythmia Suppression Trial (CAST). Am J Cardiol 76(17):1213–1217, 1995 7502998

Friedmann E, Katcher AH, Lynch JJ, Thomas SA: Animal companions and one-year survival of patients after discharge from a coronary care unit. Public Health Rep 95(4):307–312, 1980 6999524

Friedmann E, Katcher AH, Thomas SA, et al: Social interaction and blood pressure: influence of animal companions. J Nerv Ment Dis 171(8):461–465, 1983 6875529

Friedmann E, Locker BZ, Lockwood R: Perception of animals and cardiovascular responses during verbalization with an animal present. Anthrozoos 6(2):115–134, 1993

Friedmann E, Thomas SA, Son H: Pets, depression and long term survival in community living patients following myocardial infarction. Anthrozoos 24(3):273–285, 2011 21857770

Gee NR, Friedmann E, Stendahl M, et al: Heart rate variability during a working memory task: does touching a dog or person affect the response? Anthrozoos 27(4):513–528, 2014

Gee NR, Reed T, Whiting A, et al: Observing live fish improves perceptions of mood, relaxation and anxiety, but does not consistently alter heart rate or heart rate variability. Int J Environ Res Public Health 16(17):3113, 2019 31461881

Grajfoner D, Harte E, Potter LM, McGuigan N: The effect of dog-assisted intervention on student well-being, mood, and anxiety. Int J Environ Res Public Health 14(5):483, 2017 28475132

Hansen KM, Messinger CJ, Baun MM, Megel M: Companion animals alleviating distress in children. Anthrozoos 12(3):142–148, 1999

Havener L, Gentes L, Thaler B, et al: The effects of a companion animal on distress in children undergoing dental procedures. Issues Compr Pediatr Nurs 24(2):137–152, 2001 11817428

Hoffmann AO, Lee AH, Wertenauer F, et al: Dog-assisted intervention significantly reduces anxiety in hospitalized patients with major depression. Eur J Integr Med 1(3):145–148, 2009

Hoy-Gerlach J, Vincent A, Scheurmann B, Ojha M: Exploring benefits of emotional support animals (ESAs): a longitudinal pilot study with adults with serious mental illness (SMI). Hum Anim Interact Bull 10(2):1–19, 2021

Kabacoff RI, Segal DL, Hersen M, Van Hasselt VB: Psychometric properties and diagnostic utility of the Beck Anxiety Inventory and the State-Trait Anxiety Inventory with older adult psychiatric outpatients. J Anxiety Disord 11(1):33–47, 1997 9131880

Katcher AH: Interactions between people and their pets: form and function, in Interrelationships Between People and Pets. Edited by Fogle B. Springfield, IL, Charles C Thomas, 1981, pp 41–67

Katcher AH, Friedmann E, Beck AM, Lynch JJ: Talking, looking, and blood pressure: physiological consequences of interaction with the living environment, in New Perspectives on Our Lives With Animal Companions. Edited by Katcher AH, Beck AM. Philadelphia, University of Pennsylvania Press, 1983, pp 351–359

Kilpatrick DG, Resnick HS, Milanak ME, et al: National estimates of exposure to traumatic events and PTSD prevalence using DSM-IV and DSM-5 criteria. J Trauma Stress 26(5):537–547, 2013 24151000

Krause-Parello CA: Pet ownership and older women: the relationships among loneliness, pet attachment support, human social support, and depressed mood. Geriatr Nurs 33(3):194–203, 2012 22321806

Lee EH: Review of the psychometric evidence of the perceived stress scale. Asian Nurs Res (Korean Soc Nurs Sci) 6(4):121–127, 2012 25031113

Leichsenring F, Leweke F: Social anxiety disorder. N Engl J Med 376(23):2255–2264, 2017 28591542

Long JM, Lynch JJ, Machiran NM, et al: The effect of status on blood pressure during verbal communication. J Behav Med 5(2):165–172, 1982 7131540

Mueller MK, Anderson EC, King EK, Urry HL: Null effects of therapy dog interaction on adolescent anxiety during a laboratory-based social evaluative stressor. Anxiety Stress Coping 34(4):365–380, 2021 33650444

Musselman DL, Evans DL, Nemeroff CB: The relationship of depression to cardiovascular disease: epidemiology, biology, and treatment. Arch Gen Psychiatry 55(7):580–592, 1998 9672048

Nagengast SL, Baun MM, Megel M, Leibowitz JM: The effects of the presence of a companion animal on physiological arousal and behavioral distress in children during a physical examination. J Pediatr Nurs 12(6):323–330, 1997 9420370

National Institute of Mental Health: Any anxiety disorder. Bethesda, MD, National Institute of Mental Health, 2021. Available at: https://www.nimh.nih.gov/health/statistics/any-anxiety-disorder. Accessed November 28, 2021.

Nepps P, Stewart CN, Bruckno SR: Animal-assisted activity: effects of a complementary intervention program on psychological and physiological variables. J Evid Based Complementary Altern Med 19(3):211–215, 2014 24789913

O'Callaghan DM, Chandler CK: An exploratory study of animal-assisted interventions utilized by mental health professionals. J Creativity Ment Health 6(2):90–104, 2011

O'Haire ME, McKenzie SJ, Beck AM, Slaughter V: Animals may act as social buffers: skin conductance arousal in children with autism spectrum disorder in a social context. Dev Psychobiol 57(5):584–595, 2015 25913902

Orlandi M, Trangeled K, Mambrini A, et al: Pet therapy effects on oncological day hospital patients undergoing chemotherapy treatment. Anticancer Res 27(6C):4301–4303, 2007 18214035

Parslow RA, Jorm AF: Pet ownership and risk factors for cardiovascular disease: another look. Med J Aust 179(9):466–468, 2003 14583076

Pendry P, Vandagriff JL: Animal visitation program (AVP) reduces cortisol levels of university students: a randomized controlled trial. AERA Open 5(2):2332858419852592, 2019

Perez M, Cuscaden C, Somers JF, et al: Easing anxiety in preparation for pediatric magnetic resonance imaging: a pilot study using animal-assisted therapy. Pediatr Radiol 49(8):1000–1009, 2019 31030334

Polheber JP, Matchock RL: The presence of a dog attenuates cortisol and heart rate in the Trier Social Stress Test compared to human friends. J Behav Med 37(5):860–867, 2014 24170391

Rajack LS: Pets and human health: the influence of pets on cardiovascular and other aspects of owners' health. Doctoral dissertation, Cambridge, UK, University of Cambridge, 1997

Roberti JW, Harrington LN, Storch EA: Further psychometric support for the 10-item version of the perceived stress scale. J Coll Couns 9(2):135–147, 2006

Rom O, Reznick AZ: The stress reaction: a historical perspective, in Respiratory Contagion. Edited by Pokorski M. New York, Springer, 2015, pp 1–4

Rozanski A, Blumenthal JA, Kaplan J: Impact of psychological factors on the pathogenesis of cardiovascular disease and implications for therapy. Circulation 99(16):2192–2217, 1999 10217662

Salari N, Hosseinian-Far A, Jalali R, et al: Prevalence of stress, anxiety, depression among the general population during the COVID-19 pandemic: a systematic review and meta-analysis. Global Health 16(1):57, 2020 32631403

Serpell JA: Childhood pets and their influence on adults' attitudes. Psychol Rep 49(2):651–654, 1981

Shaevitz MH, Tullius JA, Callahan RT, et al: Early caregiver burden in owners of pets with suspected cancer: owner psychosocial outcomes, communication behavior, and treatment factors. J Vet Intern Med 34(6):2636–2644, 2020 32969546

Sugawara A, Masud MM, Yokoyama A, et al: Effects of presence of a familiar pet dog on regional cerebral activity in healthy volunteers: a positron emission tomography study. Anthrozoos 25(1):25–34, 2012

Tsai CC, Friedmann E, Thomas SA: The effect of animal-assisted therapy on stress responses in hospitalized children. Anthrozoos 23(3):245–258, 2010

Viau R, Arsenault-Lapierre G, Fecteau S, et al: Effect of service dogs on salivary cortisol secretion in autistic children. Psychoneuroendocrinology 35(8):1187–1193, 2010 20189722

Vogel J, Auinger A, Riedl R: Cardiovascular, neurophysiological, and biochemical stress indicators: a short review for information systems researchers, in Information Systems and Neuroscience. New York, Springer, 2019, pp 259–273

Ward-Griffin E, Klaiber P, Collins HK, et al: Petting away pre-exam stress: the effect of therapy dog sessions on student well-being. Stress Health 34(3):468–473, 2018 29528189

10

Companion Animals in the Treatment of PTSD

Cheryl A. Krause-Parello, Ph.D., R.N., FAAN
Ayse Torres, Ph.D., LMHC, CRC
Beth A. Pratt, Ph.D., R.N.
S. Juliana Moreno, B.S.N.
Sgt. David Hibler, M.S.

PTSD DEVELOPS IN SOME people who have experienced a traumatic event (National Institute of Mental Health 2017). *Trauma* is defined as any exposure to actual or threatened death, serious injury, or sexual violence (American Psychiatric Association 2022). Individuals must present with one or more symptoms lasting more than 1 month in each of the following clusters for PTSD diagnosis: trauma exposure, intrusion symptoms, avoidance, negative alterations in cognition and mood, and marked alterations in arousal and reactivity.

PTSD may develop in people after experiencing or witnessing a traumatic event, such as war, severe injury, or a serious accident (American Psychiatric Association 2022; Sareen 2021). PTSD can also develop through the indirect experience of a traumatic event, such as witnessing the interpersonal violence or a life-threatening illness of a loved one (Sareen 2021).

Prevalence of PTSD and Risk Factors

Several studies have been conducted to estimate the prevalence of PTSD in various populations. For American adult civilians, the estimated lifetime prevalence of PTSD is 6.1% (Goldstein et al. 2016), whereas among U.S. veterans, the estimated lifetime prevalence of PTSD is 9.4% (Wisco et al. 2022).

Not everyone who lives through a traumatic event develops PTSD (National Institute of Mental Health 2017). Many factors play a part in whether a person will develop PTSD. The factors that make a person more likely to develop PTSD are called *risk factors*. PTSD risk factors are generally divided into pretraumatic, peritraumatic, and posttraumatic factors.

Pretraumatic factors can be temperamental, environmental, genetic, or physiological. Pretraumatic temperamental factors include childhood emotional problems by age 6 years and previous mental disorders such as depressive disorder. Pretraumatic environmental factors include lower socioeconomic status; lower education; exposure to previous trauma; childhood adversity, such as family dysfunction; and family psychiatric history (American Psychiatric Association 2022).

Peritraumatic factors are defined as the emotional and physiological distress experienced during and/or immediately after a traumatic event and strongly predict the risk of PTSD development (Massazza et al. 2021). These factors include severity of the trauma, perceived life threat, personal injury, interpersonal violence (particularly trauma perpetrated by a caregiver), and for military personnel, the experience of witnessing atrocities or injuring someone.

Finally, *posttraumatic factors* can be temperamental or environmental. Posttraumatic temperamental factors include negative appraisals, inappropriate coping strategies, and development of acute stress disorder. Posttraumatic environmental factors include subsequent exposure to repeated upsetting reminders, subsequent adverse life events, and financial or trauma-related losses.

Clinical Presentation and Longitudinal Time Course

PTSD is characterized by intrusive thoughts related to the traumatic event, avoidance of stimuli associated with the traumatic event, negative changes in cognitions and mood, and altered arousal and anxiety (American Psychiatric Association 2022). For veterans, PTSD symptoms may manifest in many ways. Veterans may find it difficult to leave the safe confines of their home and when in public may avoid large stores, crowded spaces, or overstimulating situations that remind them of the traumatic event. They may feel like the world is always a dangerous place in which no one, even close family and friends, can be trusted. Veterans may always be on high alert, and the flight-or-fight response may be triggered when they see another person make sudden movements that mimic reaching for a weapon or when they notice debris in the middle of the road while driving that reminds them of improvised explosive devices encountered in the war zone.

PTSD symptoms follow a heterogeneous longitudinal time course. Although there has been extensive research regarding PTSD symptom trajectories, researchers have identified different trajectory classes, and have also assigned different labels to these classes. Most researchers have identified four classes of PTSD symptom trajectories over time (e.g., in military personnel and veterans [Donoho et al. 2017; Porter et al. 2017], child sexual assault survivors [Fletcher et al. 2021], and pregnant women with a history of trauma [Muzik et al. 2016]). Other researchers have identified three classes of symptom trajectories (e.g., in people who experienced whiplash [Ravn et al. 2019]) or six classes of trajectories over time (e.g., in adult residents and workers after the 2001 World Trade Center disaster [Welch et al. 2016]).

In a prospective study, Donoho et al. (2017) used latent growth mixture modeling (GMM) to determine PTSD symptom trajectory classes for a population-based representative sample of 8,178 military members from the Millennium Cohort Study. The sample included active-duty military, reservists, and national guard members. The four trajectory classes of PTSD symptoms were labeled as resilient, moderate-stable, new-onset, and preexisting. Overall, 89% of noncombat and 80% of combat military members were resilient and developed very few PTSD symptoms before, during, immediately after, and long after deployment. The moderate-stable class consisted of 7.1% noncombat and 8.6% combat military members who had slightly elevated PTSD symptoms predeployment. In the new-onset class, 2.6% of noncombat and 7.7% of combat military members had few PTSD symptoms predeployment but increased symptoms after deployment. The preexisting class, with a total of 1.2% noncombat and 3% combat military members, had the highest rate of predeployment PTSD symptoms. Current smokers, heavy drinkers, and those who experienced stressful predeployment events were more likely to be in the moderate-stable, new-onset, and preexisting trajectory classes than in the resilient class.

Porter et al. (2017) compared PTSD symptom trajectories between active-duty military members ($n = 16,788$) and veterans ($n = 5,292$) who participated in the Millennium Cohort Study by using latent GMM. Four trajectory classes were identified: delayed-onset (PTSD symptoms were low over a 3-year period and increased over the following 6-year period), improving (PTSD symptoms were high at baseline and declined over 9 years), elevated-recovering (PTSD symptoms were moderate at baseline, then increased over a 6-year period, and then declined slightly over the following 3-year period), and stable-low symptom (PTSD symptoms were low over a 9-year period). The largest number of active-duty military members (87%) and veterans (82%) were classified as being in the stable-low symptom trajectory class. More veterans were classified as part of the delayed-onset or elevated-recovering trajectory class as compared with active-duty military members, suggesting that separation from the military may be a factor in these trajectories. Although veterans tend to have higher PTSD symptomatology, veterans and active-duty personnel have similar PTSD symptom trajectories (Porter et al. 2017).

Fletcher et al. (2021) analyzed PTSD trajectories in 439 Danish child sexual assault survivors who participated in psychotherapy treatment. They used latent class growth analysis and classified four PTSD symptom trajectories of the survivors: high PTSD gradual response (high PTSD symptom levels/steady improvement response to treatment), high PTSD treatment resistant (high PTSD symptom levels/insignificant response to treatment), moderate PTSD rapid response (subclinical PTSD symptoms/rapid improvement response to treatment), and moderate PTSD gradual response (subclinical PTSD symptoms/steady improvement response to treatment). The PTSD trajectory classes were positively influenced by the amount of social support and time since the traumatic event and negatively influenced by emotional and detached coping styles, avoidance, and reexperiencing symptoms (Fletcher et al. 2021).

Muzik et al. (2016) used trajectory analysis to identify PTSD symptom trajectory categories for a population of pregnant women with lifetime PTSD (N=319). The researchers identified four distinct classes of PTSD symptom trajectories across the peripartum period: low (few symptoms), increasing (rapid symptom increase), decreasing (rapid symptom decrease), and high (slow significant symptom decline). Unlike the majority of women in the sample, approximately 26% of this population experienced an increase in PTSD symptoms during the peripartum period. The differences in this population's PTSD symptom trajectories during the peripartum period were related to their experience of stress or trauma during pregnancy, anxiety during labor, or lifetime PTSD symptoms.

Researchers have most commonly identified four PTSD symptom trajectory classes; however, other studies (Ravn et al. 2019; Welch et al.

2016) have identified different numbers of trajectory classes. Ravn et al. (2019) performed latent GMM in a prospective cohort study of people who experienced whiplash ($N=299$) and identified three PTSD symptom trajectory classes: resilient, recovering, and chronic. As with the previously mentioned studies, most individuals in this population (75.1%) were classified as resilient, with few or no PTSD symptoms over time. People in the recovering class (10%) had high initial rates of PTSD symptoms and substantial decreases in PTSD symptoms over time. However, people in the chronic class (14.9%) had high initial PTSD symptoms and a slight increase in PTSD symptoms over time. Initial pain and depression were related to the recovering and chronic classes, whereas physical pain–related disability and psychosocial pain–related disability were related to the chronic class.

Welch et al. (2016) used group-based trajectory modeling to identify six classes of PTSD symptom trajectories over time in adult residents and workers ($N=17{,}062$) after the 2001 World Trade Center disaster. The trajectory classes included low PTSD symptoms—stable over time (48.9%), moderate PTSD symptoms—stable over time (28.3%), moderate PTSD symptoms—increasing over time (8.2%), high PTSD symptoms—stable over time (6.0%), high PTSD symptoms—decreasing over time (6.6%), and very high PTSD symptoms—stable over time (2.0%). The adult residents and workers who had high levels of exposure to the disaster site, low social integration, and unemployment or job loss were more likely to have chronic, life-limiting PTSD symptoms. Regardless of the number of trajectory classes, common risk factors that appear to be associated with suboptimal trajectories include poor physical and mental health; multiple life stressors, including divorce, financial problems, sexual harassment, and disabling injury or illness; and sickness or death of a loved one.

In order for PTSD symptom management to be improved, it is important for researchers to determine a common PTSD symptom trajectory that has the potential to guide health care providers when assessing any client who has experienced a traumatic event. Screening criteria may assist the health care provider in determining frequency of assessments and interventions to cover PTSD symptom trajectories in the immediate aftermath and long after the traumatic event.

Overview of Existing Evidence-Based Treatments

Several psychological treatments for PTSD exist, including trauma-focused interventions and non-trauma-focused interventions. Trauma-focused treatments, such as prolonged exposure and cognitive processing therapy, directly address memories of the traumatic event or thoughts and feelings related to the traumatic event. Non-trauma-focused treatments, such as stress inoculation training, interpersonal therapy, and relaxation, aim to reduce PTSD symptoms, but not by directly targeting thoughts, memories, and feelings related to the traumatic event (Watkins et al. 2018).

Over the past two decades, organizations such as the American Psychological Association, National Institute for Health and Clinical Excellence, Institute of Medicine, and Veterans Health Administration/Department of Defense (VA/DoD) have produced guidelines for treatment of PTSD. Recommended treatments for PTSD are based on the most recent systematic reviews that consist of the largest and strongest evidence base available in the literature. The VA/DoD and American Psychological Association treatment guidelines published in 2017 provide the most recent recommendations for mental health practitioners who treat individuals with PTSD (American Psychological Association 2017; VA/DoD Clinical Practice Guideline Working Group 2017). These guidelines classify all treatments for adults with PTSD into two groups: "strongly recommended" and "recommended." Cognitive-behavioral therapy (CBT), cognitive processing therapy, prolonged exposure, and cognitive therapy are in the strongly recommended group. Trauma-focused CBT, cognitive processing therapy, and prolonged exposure have a substantial evidence base supporting their effectiveness in treating PTSD, although exposure-based therapies have the largest and strongest research evidence base (Cusack et al. 2016). Research and meta-analyses comparing prolonged exposure, cognitive processing therapy, and trauma-focused CBT do not find that one treatment outperforms the others (Cusack et al. 2016; Powers et al. 2010; Resick et al. 2012). The recommended treatments are eye movement desensitization therapy, brief eclectic psychotherapy, narrative exposure therapy, stress inoculation training, present-centered therapy, and interpersonal psychotherapy. Finally, the guidelines recommend several medications for the treatment of PTSD, such as sertraline, paroxetine, fluoxetine, and venlafaxine (American Psychological Association 2017; VA/DoD Clinical Practice Guideline Working Group 2017).

Although sparse, existing evidence indicates that the involvement of animal-assisted interventions (AAIs) for trauma survivors and those living with PTSD is an adjunctive treatment option to supplement usual care (e.g., medications, CBT) and to support improvements in overall health and well-being (Amerine and Hubbard 2016; Mims and Waddell 2016; O'Haire and Rodriguez 2018; Whitworth et al. 2019). Current methods of treatment include psychotherapy, counseling, and medication, but these are not always successful (Altschuler 2018; Wynn 2015). Increasing cases of PTSD in the U.S. veteran population resulting from conflicts in Iraq and Afghanistan can be difficult for clinicians to treat with the limited range of existing successful approaches (Wynn 2015). AAIs, as an alternative approach to conventional treatment, have gained popularity as a complementary treatment option to assist those living with PTSD (Amerine and Hubbard 2016; O'Haire and Rodriguez 2018; Whitworth et al. 2019; Wynn 2015). AAIs have been effective in treating a wide range of psychological conditions, such as autism, depression, anxiety, schizophrenia, and PTSD (Amerine and Hubbard 2016; Wynn 2015). Service dogs, for example, help reduce stress and anxiety, decrease blood pressure, and possibly increase oxytocin levels (Whitworth et al. 2019; Wynn 2015). Including animals as part of the treatment for PTSD in addition to conventionally successful treatment methods can be helpful in supporting beneficial outcomes, including, but not limited to, promoting a sense of comfort, motivation, and self-esteem (Amerine and Hubbard 2016). Reports have shown that AAIs significantly reduce measurable PTSD symptoms within as little as 1 week, which is much quicker in comparison to the conventional use of medication; however, a lack of rigorously acquired evidence remains (Altschuler 2018; Mims and Waddell 2016; Whitworth et al. 2019). Thus, it is crucial that AAIs continue to be explored thoroughly and urgently to better address the challenges PTSD imposes on the health and well-being of those affected.

Factors to Consider and Recommendations

Owning a service animal, an emotional support animal, or a companion dog may be a supportive addition to mental health treatments aimed at improving the owner's well-being. However, attaining a service animal comes with an abundance of obligations and financial costs for the owner (Krause-Parello et al. 2021). It is critical for mental health providers to have thoughtful discussions with their clients about the many factors to consider in service animal ownership and conduct careful evaluations of any interested client's abilities and activities.

First, owners must be able to provide the appropriate living arrangements and care for the animal's general welfare. Obtaining a service dog can carry substantial financial costs. Second, service dogs must be trained to perform their duties and to behave in public. The type of training a dog receives is dependent on the service needed by the owner. In the case of a veteran who lives with PTSD, the dog may need to be trained in emotional support to assist the veteran through panic attacks and anxiety-inducing situations (Krause-Parello et al. 2021). Searching and paying for training classes that meet the client's unique mental health needs can be difficult, especially if the owner is unable or does not know how to train the dog themselves. In addition, other factors, such as the potential effect of stress caused by the process of procuring a service dog or the owner's physical ability to exercise, should be considered.

Providers should be aware of their clients' lifestyle preferences and limits in regard to their physical, mental, and emotional capabilities in order to assess their ability to care for an animal. An animal that can live a healthy life in alignment with the owner's lifestyle is most beneficial for a client seeking therapeutic benefits from owning a dog. For instance, a veteran with PTSD who may have previously owned a dog when they were younger and is seeking to own a companion dog now has trouble walking for long periods of time. Considering this, a provider should become informed on the different types of dogs that are best suited for the veteran client (Krause-Parello et al. 2021).

In order to practically provide care for their clients, providers should thoughtfully consider aspects of their health that affect their daily lives. It is crucial to inform and educate clients on their personal role in the maintenance of owning an animal, because it is a significant choice that affects the lives of both the client and the animal. For instance, companion dogs do not require any prescription from a provider; however, providers should inform their clients of the responsibilities inherent in providing for their dog, such as training or certification.

Ownership of the animal comes with a variety of secondary details that must be evaluated to ensure the well-being of both the client and the animal. These details include, but are not limited to, having sufficient financial means to responsibly provide for the animal's veterinary health care, pet insurance, food, training, grooming, and other associated costs. Some properties may have restrictions or fees that can be a potential barrier to owning an animal. Although animals offer helpful support and their owners do have the right to protect themselves, property owners can still enforce certain rules regarding animals living on the property (Humane Society of the United States 2021). It is not expected that a provider understand the exact specifications of each client's living circumstances; however, having the capacity and knowledge to educate clients on the possible obstacles associated with animals living on a property is a valuable service that can better prepare their clients for owning an animal. It is important for a provider to follow up and check on the health of both the animal and the client as they adapt to adjustments that must be made. The health of one will affect that of the other, so attention to both should be consistent in supporting the therapeutic bond between the client and the animal (Krause-Parello et al. 2021).

Quality and Strength of Existing Evidence Supporting Animal-Assisted Interventions

Human-animal interaction (HAI) is a relatively new field of study compared with other, more mature fields. For this fairly new area of inquiry, the quality of the research is an important aspect to consider. An investigator's methodological approach and research design affect the rigor of the evidence. Randomized controlled trials (RCTs; single-, double-, or triple-blind) are considered the gold standard in research design. In an attempt to reduce bias, this methodology supports random assignment to a condition, an intervention, or a comparison or control condition. However, it may be difficult to design HAI research that is blinded for obvious reasons. There is a dearth of RCTs in the field of HAI, especially for studies on PTSD. However, well-designed RCTs do exist. One randomized controlled study investigated the preliminary efficacy (O'Haire and Rodriguez 2018) and others examined the significance (LaFollette et al. 2019; Rodriguez et al. 2020, 2021) of service dogs for veterans with PTSD.

Some studies that investigated the involvement of animals with the goal of reducing PTSD symptom severity use terms to describe the research design such as pilot, feasibility, proof of concept, and preliminary efficacy. When evaluating the quality of these types of studies, one must bear in mind that methodological challenges frequently exist. Sample sizes are often relatively small and may include a homogeneous population lacking diversity (e.g., ethnicity and race), and consequently the findings will not be generalizable to the population at large. In addition, the information needed to calculate effect size and conduct a power analysis may be missing; this lack of information limits other researchers when they attempt to ascertain meaningful associations between the variables being studied or the differences between the groups.

There are various theoretical frameworks that can be used in studies on the effect of AAIs in patients with PTSD. The biopsychosocial model (Engel 1977) is used most frequently to guide current HAI studies on the involvement of animals in the treatment of PTSD (Gee et al. 2021). An example of the questions researchers frequently ask is: Are AAIs associated with reductions in PTSD symptoms and related sequelae (e.g., reductions in depression, suicidal ideation, anxiety)?

Based on a review of existing evidence, the animals most commonly involved in interventions for PTSD are dogs. However, other animals are represented, including horses (Johnson et al. 2018; Monroe et al. 2019). This makes it difficult to know all the animals that may be effective and what type of animal is most effective for whom and under what circumstances.

In some more established or mature disciplines, funding for scientific inquiry is abundant. Unfortunately, limited funding sources are available for conducting HAI research (Serpell 2012). This is unfortunate because the researchers in this field compete against one another for resources, thus restraining the growth of the field in comparison to others.

Case Example (Sgt. David Hibler, M.S.)

I was an army combat medic; I understand how the military can take a toll on veterans. While in Iraq, I saw how relationships with animals could help mitigate that toll. Many of these relationships, especially with dogs, brought significant opportunities for healing.

In Iraq, I was posted near a zoo that Saddam Hussein kept. Because of this, there were many strays around, especially dogs and cats. Official guidance was to stay clear of them for health and safety, but many of these animals ended up becoming unit "mascots." These animals became so important that many soldiers went through the long, costly process of quarantining and shipping them home. The connections that soldiers formed with these animals would often be as strong as connections with other members of their units.

Orion is my dog. He was prescribed to me to help with posttraumatic stress and transition back to civilian life. When it was first suggested that a dog would help with transitioning home, I didn't see how it could. But I have been astonished by how much Orion has helped me.

When I returned, I found that a lot of deployment stress had followed me home. I would stay up late with restless thoughts. Sometimes I would oversocialize or imbibe to de-stress. Then the following day, I would often be tired or have trouble functioning. I started losing my ability to keep a schedule. I never realized how important keeping a schedule is. It can make or break your day, and with enough bad days your life can fall into disarray.

This hurt me in multiple ways. Physically, I was stressed, I wasn't as active, and my blood pressure and cholesterol were rising. Socially I was unreliable, romantic relationships became unstable, relationships with family and friends were strained, and my university grade point average had fallen to 2.1 on a 4.0 scale. Psychologically, I wasn't sleeping well; I was diagnosed with PTSD, depression, and anxiety; and I was losing purpose. My postcombat stress was dismantling my life, and my health was cratering as a result.

It wasn't immediate, but Orion helped me with all these issues. He keeps me active, and my cholesterol and blood pressure have improved.

Having him forced me into a structured schedule and required me to be responsible with my time. This structure helps with keeping track of responsibilities, and my grade point average is now 3.7. Having a consistent schedule allowed me to become a more reliable person, stable romantic partner, and better friend. My relationships are healthier now thanks to the meta-effect Orion has had on my life.

Having Orion helps me sleep better. He gives me a sense of security and, if I'm up late, a look that says, "It's bedtime." Having him also requires me to wake up on time to feed and let him out. Knowing that I am responsible to get home and take care of him helps me keep my day in order and gives me purpose.

More so than just a schedule, he helps me with deeper things that can be hard to explain. One of the most difficult parts of coming home was not having my battle buddies around, just being alone in the dark and quiet. That is when depression can really grab you. It feels like you are sinking into a bottomless hole. With Orion around, it doesn't feel that bad. He helps to mitigate my PTSD, depression, and anxiety. Sometimes it's the physical contact of petting him, sometimes it's talking to him, and sometimes it's just knowing that he's there. It is hard to say exactly what it is every time, but just having a dog there can make a big difference for a veteran who is dealing with an invisible attack like that.

Additionally, having someone who relies on you gives a certain element of purpose. Purpose is something military personnel have in excess while they are serving. However, when your duty is done, many veterans feel a lack of purpose to their lives. Without that purpose, some veterans conclude that their lives lack meaning and are not worth the difficulties plaguing them. Having a dog who relies on you helps to establish a foothold for veterans that reminds them how important and purposeful their lives are.

Orion is 14 now. He is old and having health issues, but he is still my closest friend. He has been there for me in ways I don't think I could have asked of another person. Some scars will never go away, but Orion has helped me heal significantly. I have seen how much these animals mean to soldiers during war, and I have been lucky to experience how much they help us afterward.

Key Clinical Points

- Before recommending a service animal, emotional support animal, or companion animal for a client with PTSD, the clinician must conduct careful evaluations of the client's abilities and interests.

- The clinician must consider animal welfare by determining the client's ability to care for the animal financially and physically and to provide the necessary time for training.

- Before recommending a service dog, a clinician must assess factors such as the potential effect of stress caused by the process of procuring a service dog as well as the owner's physical ability to exercise.

References

Altschuler EL: Animal-assisted therapy for post-traumatic stress disorder: lessons from "case reports" in media stories. Mil Med 183(1–2):11–13, 2018 29401355

American Psychiatric Association: Diagnostic and Statistical Manual of Mental Disorders, 5th Edition, Text Revision. Washington, DC, American Psychiatric Association, 2022

American Psychological Association: Clinical Practice Guideline for the Treatment of Posttraumatic Stress Disorder (PTSD) in Adults. Washington, DC, American Psychological Association, 2017

Amerine JL, Hubbard GB: Using animal-assisted therapy to enrich psychotherapy. Adv Mind Body Med 30(3):11, 2016 27541053

Cusack K, Jonas DE, Forneris CA, et al: Psychological treatments for adults with posttraumatic stress disorder: a systematic review and meta-analysis. Clin Psychol Rev 43:128–141, 2016 26574151

Donoho CJ, Bonanno GA, Porter B, et al: A decade of war: prospective trajectories of posttraumatic stress disorder symptoms among deployed US military personnel and the influence of combat exposure. Am J Epidemiol 186(12):1310–1318, 2017 29036483

Engel GL: The need for a new medical model: a challenge for biomedicine. Science 196(4286):129–136, 1977 847460

Fletcher S, Elklit A, Shevlin M, Armour C: Predictors of PTSD treatment response trajectories in a sample of childhood sexual abuse survivors: the roles of social support, coping, and PTSD symptom clusters. J Interpers Violence 36(3–4):1283–1307, 2021 29294985

Gee NR, Rodriguez KE, Fine AH, Trammell JP: Dogs supporting human health and well-being: a biopsychosocial approach. Front Vet Sci 8:630465, 2021 33860004

Goldstein RB, Smith SM, Chou SP, et al: The epidemiology of DSM-5 posttraumatic stress disorder in the United States: results from the National Epidemiologic Survey on Alcohol and Related Conditions-III. Soc Psychiatry Psychiatr Epidemiol 51(8):1137–1148, 2016

Humane Society of the United States: Information for renters with pets. Washington, DC, Humane Society of the United States, 2021. Available at: https://www.humanesociety.org/resources/information-renters-pets. Accessed August 1, 2021.

Johnson RA, Albright DL, Marzolf JR, et al: Effects of therapeutic horseback riding on post-traumatic stress disorder in military veterans. Mil Med Res 5(1):3, 2018 29502529

Krause-Parello CA, Boyrer AE, Moreno SJ, Meyer E: The use of service, emotional support, and companion animals as a complementary health approach for military veterans: information for healthcare providers, in Caring for Veterans and Their Families: A Guide for Nurses and Other Healthcare Professionals. Edited by D'Aoust RF, Rossiter AG. Burlington, MA, Jones and Bartlett, 2021, pp 139–151

LaFollette MR, Rodriguez KE, Ogata N, O'Haire ME: Military veterans and their PTSD service dogs: associations between training methods, PTSD severity, dog behavior, and the human-animal bond. Front Vet Sci 6:23, 2019 30805353

Massazza A, Joffe H, Hyland P, Brewin CR: The structure of peritraumatic reactions and their relationship with PTSD among disaster survivors. J Abnorm Psychol 130(3):248–259, 2021 33539115

Mims D, Waddell R: Animal assisted therapy and trauma survivors. J Evid Inf Soc Work 13(5):452–457, 2016 27210487

Monroe M, Whitworth JD, Wharton T, Turner J: Effects of an equine-assisted therapy program for military veterans with self-reported PTSD. Soc Anim 29(5–6):577–590, 2019

Muzik M, McGinnis EW, Bocknek E, et al: PTSD symptoms across pregnancy and early postpartum among women with lifetime PTSD diagnosis. Depress Anxiety 33(7):584–591, 2016 26740305

National Institute of Mental Health: Post-traumatic stress disorder. Bethesda, MD, National Institute of Mental Health, 2017. Available at: https://www.nimh.nih.gov/health/topics/post-traumatic-stress-disorder-ptsd/#part_145372. Accessed June 12, 2021.

O'Haire ME, Rodriguez KE: Preliminary efficacy of service dogs as a complementary treatment for posttraumatic stress disorder in military members and veterans. J Consult Clin Psychol 86(2):179–188, 2018 29369663

Porter B, Bonanno GA, Frasco MA, et al: Prospective post-traumatic stress disorder symptom trajectories in active duty and separated military personnel. J Psychiatr Res 89:55–64, 2017 28182961

Powers MB, Halpern JM, Ferenschak MP, et al: A meta-analytic review of prolonged exposure for posttraumatic stress disorder. Clin Psychol Rev 30(6):635–641, 2010 20546985

Ravn SL, Karstoft KI, Sterling M, Andersen TE: Trajectories of posttraumatic stress symptoms after whiplash: a prospective cohort study. Eur J Pain 23(3):515–525, 2019 30318773

Resick PA, Williams LF, Suvak MK, et al: Long-term outcomes of cognitive-behavioral treatments for posttraumatic stress disorder among female rape survivors. J Consult Clin Psychol 80(2):201–210, 2012 22182261

Rodriguez KE, LaFollette MR, Hediger K, et al: Defining the PTSD service dog intervention: perceived importance, usage, and symptom specificity of psychiatric service dogs for military veterans. Front Psychol 11:1638, 2020 32849004

Rodriguez KE, Anderson LM, Ott CA, O'Haire ME: The effect of a PTSD service dog on military veterans' medication regimens: a cross-sectional pilot study. Anthrozoos 34(3):393–406, 2021 34140755

Sareen J: Posttraumatic stress disorder in adults: epidemiology, pathophysiology, clinical manifestations, course, assessment, and diagnosis. UpToDate, 2021. Available at: https://www.uptodate.com/contents/posttraumatic-stress-disorder-in-adults-epidemiology-pathophysiology-clinical-manifestations-course-assessment-and-diagnosis. Accessed August 2, 2021.

Serpell J: Foreword, in Waltham Pocket Book of Human-Animal Interactions. Buckinghamshire, England, Beyond Design Solutions, 2012

VA/DoD Clinical Practice Guideline Working Group: VA/DoD Clinical Practice Guideline for the Management of Posttraumatic Stress Disorder and Acute Stress Disorder. Washington, DC, VA Office of Quality and Performance, 2017

Watkins LE, Sprang KR, Rothbaum BO: Treating PTSD: a review of evidence-based psychotherapy interventions. Front Behav Neurosci 12:258, 2018 30450043

Welch AE, Caramanica K, Maslow CB, et al: Trajectories of PTSD among lower Manhattan residents and area workers following the 2001 World Trade Center disaster, 2003–2012. J Trauma Stress 29(2):158–166, 2016 26954702

Whitworth JD, Scotland-Coogan D, Wharton T: Service dog training programs for veterans with PTSD: results of a pilot controlled study. Soc Work Health Care 58(4):412–430, 2019 30875483

Wisco BE, Nomamiukor FO, Marx BP, et al: Posttraumatic stress disorder in US military veterans: results from the 2019-2020 National Health and Resilience in Veterans Study. J Clin Psychiatry 83(2):20m14029, 2022 35192748

Wynn GH: Complementary and alternative medicine approaches in the treatment of PTSD. Curr Psychiatry Rep 17(8):600, 2015 26073362

11

Companion Animals in the Treatment of Serious Mental Illness

Lisa D. Townsend, Ph.D., LCSW
Peter F. Buckley, M.D.

NONAFFECTIVE PSYCHOTIC illnesses, such as schizophrenia, form the main focus of this chapter. Collectively, we refer to them as *serious mental illness* (SMI), although most research has been done with regard to schizophrenia specifically. We provide key insights from the human-animal interaction (HAI) literature on the role that animals may play in facilitating recovery for people with SMI. There is substantial variability in how HAI terms are used. In order to promote greater clarity and consistency in the HAI field, in this chapter we use the following terms adapted from an International Association of Human-Animal Interaction Organizations (2018) white paper: 1) animal-assisted activities (AAAs)—informal HAIs conducted for motivational, educational, or recreational purposes; 2) animal-assisted interventions (AAIs)—goal-oriented and structured interventions incorporating animals into therapeutic services; and 3) animal-assisted therapy (AAT)—goal-oriented and structured therapeutic interventions that are planned and delivered by health or education professionals.

Prevalence of Serious Mental Illness and Risk Factors

Although statistically rare (0.3%–0.5% of the U.S. population; Kessler et al. 2005; Wu et al. 2006), psychotic illnesses are among the most debilitating disorders, with increased risk of morbidity (Olfson et al. 2015) and mortality (Palmer et al. 2005).

Multiple factors are believed to confer risk for schizophrenia. These include genetic and environmental factors and, most likely, interaction between the two (van de Leemput et al. 2016). Current scientific thinking suggests that schizophrenia results from a complex interplay between genetics, epigenetic changes, and environmental exposures. Environmental risks range from prenatal and birth insults (Brown and Meyer 2018; Jones et al. 1998; Opler et al. 2013; Pugliese et al. 2019) to family conflict (Bebbington and Kuipers 1994; Finnegan et al. 2014) and poverty (Johnson et al. 1999; Newbury et al. 2022).

Clinical Presentation and Longitudinal Time Course

Schizophrenia is characterized by hallucinations and/or delusions, along with cognitive and motivational disturbances, such as difficulty processing information and poor hygiene. People who have schizophrenia often struggle with daily life activities, such as keeping up with hygiene and maintaining a household, and have difficulties sustaining regular employment. They frequently experience barriers to developing and maintaining social relationships. Social networks in this population are often composed primarily of family members and contain proportionately fewer friends than the social networks of people without SMI (Palumbo et al. 2015). Symptoms of schizophrenia are pervasive and persistent, affecting educational and employment opportunities as well as social functioning throughout the life course.

Overview of Evidence-Based Treatments for Schizophrenia

Evidence-based treatment for schizophrenia typically involves antipsychotic medications along with psychosocial and community supports. Treatment can be undermined by noncompliance with medications, which can have high rates of side effects, including oversedation, metabolic disturbances, and obesity. Therapeutic supports for people with schizophrenia include case management, supportive housing, and employment or educational services, with case management serving as a cornerstone of community-based treatment for SMI (Adamou 2005).

Role of Animals in Supporting People With Serious Mental Illness

A variety of AAAs and AAIs and types of AAT have been explored as adjunctive treatments for schizophrenia. Such interventions range from animal visitation on inpatient or residential units to more immersive, experiential therapies that teach coping or occupational skills. The primary goal of AAIs and AAT is to address deficits in motivation, communication, and social engagement. Some research indicates that AAIs and AAT also may reduce positive symptoms. Treatment involving animals is designed to augment standard pharmacological and psychosocial interventions, not to replace them. Therapeutic activities range in complexity from interacting temporarily with a visiting animal and their handler to learning to ride a horse and participating in farmwork.

Therapeutic outcomes addressed by AAIs and AAT include negative symptoms of schizophrenia, such as poverty of speech or amotivation, and basic social and psychological targets, such as self-efficacy, self-confidence, and social skills, as well as social communication and aggression. Hypothesized mechanisms by which AAIs and AAT affect outcomes include social mediation (animals facilitate conversations between people), facilitation of self-efficacy (animals assist in skill acquisition), attachment (patients build relationships with animals who may serve as attachment figures), and physiological effects (improved physical health through exercise, anxiety reduction via upregulation of the parasympathetic nervous system) (Berget and Braastad 2008). This mechanistic framework is consistent with the biopsychosocial model of human behavior, which accounts for the dynamic interplay between internal physical, cognitive, and emotional processes, as well as environmental influences (Gee et al. 2021).

Understanding the Types of Animal-Assisted Interventions Used in Populations With Serious Mental Illness

Interventions vary in terms of structure, complexity, length, frequency, and types of animals involved. The animals most commonly involved in treatment programs for people with schizophrenia are horses and dogs, but programs are not restricted to just two types of animals. For example, one of the most complex experiential interventions is Green Care, which includes AAIs with a variety of farm animals, horticultural therapy, or simply basic farmwork (Artz and Bitler Davis 2017). The common underlying feature of Green Care programs involves interaction with nature to achieve a therapeutic goal. Some programs also incorporate regular interactions with farm staff to foster socialization (Berget and Braastad 2011). Patients participating in such programs receive training in farmwork and animal care and potential opportunities for ongoing volunteer work or paid employment. Green Care has been more widely implemented in Europe than in the United States because of the lack of studies regarding its efficacy and corresponding lack of insurance coverage.

Horses are frequently involved in Green Care and other types of AAIs and AAT. Equine therapy organizations, such as the Equine Assisted Growth and Learning Association (EAGALA; www.eagala.org) and Professional Association of Therapeutic Horsemanship International (PATH International; www.pathintl.org), have developed curricula to guide therapeutic interventions for various patient populations. EAGALA pairs a licensed mental health professional with an equine specialist to achieve specific therapeutic goals through structured interactions with horses. PATH International offers similar therapeutic activities while incorporating mounted exercises. Interventions are conducted individually and with groups and are made up of activities such as grooming or guiding a horse through an obstacle course hands-free. Reflective activities ask patients to consider how the horses respond to their behaviors and how these insights translate to their daily lives and relationships.

AAT involving dogs has typically been implemented in residential or inpatient settings. Many interventions involve patients interacting with a dog during structured group therapy. Therapeutic activities range from petting and talking to the dog to training the dog to do tricks or perform a series of activities.

Involving Resident Animals in the Treatment of Schizophrenia

Many people with schizophrenia require long-term residential care. One way that animals are involved in caring for people in residential treatment is to enhance or normalize the social milieu. Involving a resident animal can create a sense of home and normalcy while fostering social interactions. Research indicates that most patients and staff welcome animals on residential units and perceive significant benefits from their presence. Patient and staff self-report data suggest that "ward" animals are seen as welcome additions to an inpatient unit (Wagner et al. 2019). Surveys and semistructured interviews with 33 psychiatric inpatients with depression ($n=20$) or psychosis ($n=13$) and staff members on wards with and without a resident cat measured attitudes toward having a residential cat and beliefs about the cat's effect on the inpatient atmosphere, their social interactions, and well-being. Overall, staff and patients reported positive attitudes toward ward cats. All patients on the unit with the ward cat reported that the cat was associated with positive effects, and all but one preferred a unit with a cat.

Birds also have been included in efforts to normalize residential treatment environments and motivate patients to engage in caregiving activities and social interactions. Seventy male inpatients in residential care homes were randomly assigned to a control group (no intervention) or an AAA involving caring for a pet bird for 8 weeks. Results indicated a significant increase in happiness and quality of life for the AAA group compared with the control group (Sahebalzamani et al. 2020).

Addressing Positive and Negative Symptoms of Schizophrenia

Positive symptoms of schizophrenia (hallucinations, delusions), as well as negative ones (anhedonia, inactivity), interfere with individuals' ability to engage in employment, education, self-care, and recreation. As outlined at the beginning of this section, standard treatment involves medication and supportive services. However, randomized controlled trials suggest that adjunctive AAT confers additional symptom reduction benefits. Calvo et al. (2016) randomly assigned 22 adults with schizophrenia to two 1-hour weekly AAT groups with a dog or a control condition in the context of a residential psychiatric rehabilitation program. Both groups received standard elements of psychiatric rehabilitation, which included individual psychotherapy, group therapy, programming to improve daily functioning, community reintegration services, and family work. The control group received weekly group therapy that included one non-AAT activity designed to improve daily functioning. Therapy activities in the AAT group included emotional bonding work between patients and the dog (grooming and taking care of the dog), dog walking, and dog training or play. Even though both groups had a significant decrease in positive symptoms of schizophrenia, the AAT group also experienced significant decreases in negative symptoms, which are more challenging to treat, and greater adherence to therapy sessions.

Anhedonia is a common negative symptom associated with psychotic illnesses and is often intransigent and particularly treatment refractory. Anhedonic presentation may include poverty of speech, difficulty completing personal hygiene, and lack of motivation. AAT with a dog may play a role in ameliorating its debilitating effects. Nathans-Barel et al. (2005) allocated 20 long-term inpatients with schizophrenia to 10 weeks of once-weekly individual AAT with a dog or treatment as usual. Primary outcome anhedonia scores were significantly improved in the AAT group; AAT participants also showed significantly increased leisure activities following the intervention.

Taken together, these studies provide support for AAT as an augmentation of standard treatment for positive and negative symptoms of schizophrenia. Furthermore, there may be a specific benefit to involving animals in their ability to address intractable negative symptoms that are difficult to treat with other methods.

Improving Social Interactions and Communication

Even when primary symptoms are well managed, patients who have schizophrenia often struggle with stigma, social exclusion, and lack of desire to form social relationships. Studies examining social interaction outcomes suggest that involving animals may break down barriers to patients' engagement with other people (Berget and Braastad 2008). Reviews of Green Care programs generally support the efficacy of these treatments for enhancing social communication skills and indicate that patients derive a strong sense of social support from their farm experiences (Berget and Braastad 2011; Jormfeldt and Carlsson 2018).

Less complex interventions also have been associated with improvements in social communication for patients. Ten participants with SMI in long-term nursing home care participated in a group intervention that evaluated pre- and postintervention communication behaviors using an A/B design that controlled for novelty effects. The intervention used a 2-week handler-only condition followed by a 14-week handler-plus-dog intervention, ending with 2 weeks of observation only (Hall and Malpus 2000). Both verbal and nonverbal behaviors increased during the handler-plus-dog intervention compared with the other conditions. Communication levels decreased again during the 2-week posttreatment observation period, suggesting that if the association between the canine-assisted intervention and the social communication benefits is causal, ongoing interaction with the handler/dog team may be required for sustained improvement.

Enhancing Self-Efficacy and Coping Skills

Self-efficacy and general coping skills form the foundation for engaging in routine and novel activities and managing daily stress; these qualities are frequently compromised in people with schizophrenia. AAIs may enhance patients' sense of capability and coping with daily stressors according to a review of 13 quantitative and qualitative studies involving Green Care programs (Berget and Braastad 2011). Findings specific to people with SMI indicated that care farming was associated with increases in self-efficacy for this population.

Beyond self-efficacy, AAIs are associated with improvements in coping and perceived quality of life among people with SMI. Berget et al. (2008) investigated the efficacy of work with farm animals and Green Care among 14 inpatients and 76 outpatients with a variety of diagnoses, including psychotic illness. All patients received psychotherapy and medication as part of their regular treatment; some patients were randomly assigned to participate in an adjunctive Green Care AAI. The AAI group visited a farm twice a week for 12 weeks to work with the animals. Findings indicated a significant improvement in self-efficacy, coping, and quality of life in the AAI group compared with control subjects. Gains became apparent from the end of the treatment period to the 6-month follow-up, suggesting that the effects of AAI accrue over time and are sustained at least in the short-term.

Similar benefits have been seen with programs that involve dogs. Weekly 50-minute group AAI sessions, in a trial lasting for 8 weeks, were associated with improvements in some psychological symptoms in 30 Taiwanese inpatients with schizophrenia (Chu et al. 2009). Patients were randomly assigned to participate in structured AAI sessions with dogs that included petting the dogs, playing fetch, and walking the dogs through an obstacle course. Self-report outcome measures were collected 1 week before and 1 week after the 8-week intervention. Significant improvements were found for self-esteem, self-determination, positive psychotic symptoms, and emotional symptoms but not for social support and negative symptoms.

Improving Mood and Reducing Anxiety

Low mood and anxiety frequently accompany positive and negative symptoms of schizophrenia. Just as in people without SMI, people with psychotic illness may experience anxiolytic effects of animals. In a study by Seredova et al. (2016), group hippotherapy (therapy involving horses) was evaluated among 25 inpatients. Patients received 90 minutes of therapy twice weekly for 3 weeks. Significant improvements were found in patient self-report measures of well-being, mood, and tension but not in self-report measures of fear, willingness to make social connections, and willingness to communicate.

A pre-post crossover study conducted with 14 inpatients struggling with acute exacerbations of schizophrenia reported reductions in anxiety during conversational interviews when a dog was involved compared with similar sessions without a dog (Lang et al. 2010). Patients received a 30-minute interview about pets and animal-related topics with a research assistant only or an interaction with the research assistant and a dog. Interventions were counterbalanced and occurred over 2 consecutive days. Findings indicated significant reductions in state anxiety in the presence of a dog compared with the presence of a person only.

Although additional studies are needed to replicate and extend these initial findings, results indicate that hippotherapy and canine-assisted interventions may have anxiolytic effects. Additionally, findings from Lang et al. (2010) illustrated the potential of animals to facilitate psychiatric interviews with anxious patients, possibly because the animal's presence sets the stage for a more empathetic form of interaction.

Managing Activities of Daily Living and Self-Care

Managing daily tasks such as finances, cleaning, and personal hygiene poses significant challenges to people living with schizophrenia and is a frequent intervention target for case management. Studies suggest that AAIs may play a role in sparking engagement in these activities. Kovács et al. (2004) recruited seven long-term inpatients with schizophrenia to participate in a 9-month group therapy program involving a dog. Therapeutic tasks included greeting the dog, grooming, physical exercise, and cooperative group activities. Outcome measures included seven domains from the Independent Living Skills Survey, which assesses daily behaviors related to eating, personal hygiene, domestic activities, health, money management, transportation, and leisure activities. Findings showed significant improvements in completion of domestic activities and in health. All patients participated consistently in the therapy program with no attrition.

Reducing Aggressive Behavior

One of the most concerning aspects of psychotic illnesses is the presence of aggressive behavior, particularly when patients are experiencing intense psychotic symptoms or agitation. Aggressive behavior may not respond thoroughly or immediately to psychosocial interventions, necessitating pharmacological intervention. However, evidence exists that hippotherapy is associated with reductions in violent behavior in people with psychotic illnesses. Ninety long-term inpatients (mean = 5.4 years) were randomly assigned to one of four weekly groups: 1) equine-assisted psychotherapy, 2) canine-assisted psychotherapy, 3) enhanced social skills therapy (active control), or 4) regular hospital care (inactive control; Nurenberg et al. 2015). The primary outcome measure was violence-related incident reports, collected for 2 months before treatment and for 3 months after treatment initiation. The equine-assisted therapy group used the EAGALA model and involved groundwork only. An example activity involved leading a horse in a designated pattern through a series of cones. Equine-assisted psychotherapy was significantly associated with decreases in violent incident reports; violent incidents actually increased in the other three groups. Although this study suggests that equine therapy may be helpful for reducing aggressive behavior, it also serves as a caution when one is considering involving dogs in similar treatments.

Patient and Staff Perceptions of Interactions With Animals

Intervention acceptability is a vital prerequisite to establishing a successful AAI program. Studies examining patient and staff reactions to AAIs provide encouraging evidence of program acceptability. Semi-structured interviews were completed with community-dwelling patients with schizophrenia or schizoaffective disorder before and after a 10-week hippotherapy intervention (Corring et al. 2013). Themes included 1) having fun (one patient noted freedom from hallucinations during and after riding); 2) bonding with the horses; 3) increasing confidence and self-esteem; 4) experiencing improvements in relationships with other humans; and 5) increasing staff realization that patients had greater potential than was previously acknowledged and required less protection. Some studies with random assignment of patients to AAT versus comparator groups reported reduced or no attrition in AAT study arms (Berget et al. 2008; Calvo et al. 2016). Similarly, evaluations of staff receptivity to resident animals or AAI programming indicated that staff welcome these interventions (Abrahamson et al. 2016; Sallette et al. 2021).

Role of Robotic Animals

Although most interventions have been conducted with living animals, there may be a role for robotic animals under conditions that are infeasible or unsafe for live ones. AIBO is a robotic dog that can be "trained" to perform a series of behaviors, such as playing fetch (Narita et al. 2016). Participants in a pilot study involving AIBO included three Japanese long-term inpatients who had schizophrenia. The intervention involved weekly hourlong interactions with AIBO for 8 weeks. Findings indicated decreases in anxiety, depressive symptoms, motor retardation, emotional withdrawal, and avoidance of social interactions. The same authors used a single-case-study design to evaluate mental health outcomes with a female Japanese patient with schizophrenia. She received 8 weeks of weekly 1-hour therapy with AIBO. At the end of the 8 weeks, anxiety, depression, and motor retardation scores decreased by approximately half. Current mechanistic theories posit that therapeutic benefits are dependent on the mutuality inherent in interactions between living beings, so further research is needed on the role of artificial intelligence in supporting people with schizophrenia. However, robotic animals may serve as a proxy if safety and animal welfare considerations preclude AAIs.

Companion Animals and Schizophrenia

Although much of the research presented earlier relates to AAIs, some research has evaluated the roles that companion animals (pets) play in the lives of people with SMI. Qualitative interviews with four people diagnosed with SMI identified themes about the role of companion animals in their recovery (Wisdom et al. 2009). Diagnoses included schizophrenia, schizoaffective disorder, bipolar illness, and affective psychosis. Four themes were synthesized: 1) pets provided empathy and were seen as therapeutic; 2) pets either served as social connections themselves or facilitated social interactions with other people; 3) pets served as surrogate family members; and 4) pets supported self-efficacy and empowerment. Some interviewees reported feeling at times overwhelmed by caring for their pets and experiencing mental health setbacks related to pet loss. Collaborative programs have explored connecting people with SMI living in community-based housing with shelter animals. Early findings suggest that adopting a shelter animal may be associated with improvements in anxiety, depression, and loneliness (Hoy-Gerlach et al. 2021).

When the appropriateness of a companion animal for community-dwelling patients is being assessed, it is vital to evaluate whether the individual can provide a stable, calm environment for the animal long-term. Other considerations include adequate income to support the animal's care, transportation for veterinary care, and low risk of aggressive behavior toward the animal. It may be important to establish a designee who cares for the companion animal if a patient experiences symptom exacerbation or hospitalization.

Clinical and Animal Welfare Considerations

Screening patients before involving them in AAT is highly recommended. Patients with schizophrenia or schizoaffective disorder completed surveys regarding their opinions of animals in general as well as involving them in treatment (Iwahashi et al. 2007). More than 80% of patients reported liking animals; however, only 57% thought that therapy animals would be a useful addition to their psychiatric care. Screening is critical for determining whether patients like interacting with animals and whether they can do so safely. This is especially important for group AAT and residential/facility animals. Chandler (2012) developed a screening form to evaluate patients' appropriateness for participating in AAT. Assessment questions include fears of animals, allergies, desire to participate in AAT, and history of aggression toward people or animals. Lastly, it is vital that animals involved in AAIs have a designated advocate to protect their well-being.

Quality and Strength of Evidence for Animal-Assisted Interventions in Treating Serious Mental Illness

Meta-analyses and systematic reviews can effectively summarize the state of the science regarding interventions for a given condition. Unfortunately, studies of AAAs, AAIs, and AAT for schizophrenia and psychotic illnesses suffer from significant heterogeneity (Hawkins et al. 2019), and few meta-analytic studies have been conducted. Interventions vary widely in terms of the types of animals involved, therapeutic modalities, and outcome measures, leading to difficulty drawing global conclusions about the efficacy of HAIs for schizophrenia and related illnesses.

A systematic review of six Green Care–based equine-assisted therapy studies for adults with schizophrenia suggested that equine-assisted therapy has potential for reducing negative symptoms and improving self-confidence, decreasing the need for emergency and long-term care, and reducing aggressive behavior among inpatients (Jormfeldt and Carlsson 2018). A range of intervention and therapy activities, such as bonding with the horses, stable work, and horseback riding, were used in these studies. Greater consistency in intervention structure, the types of animals involved, and outcome measures would allow firmer conclusions to be drawn regarding AAIs and AAT for people with schizophrenia and form a foundation for tailoring interventions to address specific symptoms or target outcomes.

Areas for Future Research

Most AAI studies conducted with individuals who have schizophrenia have measured short-term outcomes. For those studies that have had promising results, longer-term measurement periods are needed to assess whether mental health improvements are sustained. Along the same lines, it would be useful to know whether AAIs have dosage effects—for example, is once weekly for an hour enough to stimulate improvements, or could faster or greater improvement be achieved by increasing interaction frequency?

Likewise, most studies of AAIs have been conducted with inpatients, many of whom were long-term residents of a psychiatric hospital. It would be helpful to replicate those positive study findings with outpatients to determine whether AAIs can play a role in preventing repeat hospitalizations.

From a research design standpoint, tightening of methodology would advance the field; for example, reducing heterogeneity in study samples and increasing sample sizes would go a long way toward enabling stronger conclusions to be drawn regarding AAIs for schizophrenia. Finally, manualized, theoretically grounded, empirically evaluated, and reproducible interventions are clearly needed to provide consistency of delivery and predictability of outcomes.

Case Example

Ms. K, a 45-year-old woman, was diagnosed with schizoaffective disorder and PTSD. She frequently uses inpatient psychiatric treatment when her moods destabilize or she experiences exacerbations of her psychosis.

She receives case management through an Assertive Community Treatment (ACT) team along with outpatient psychiatry and psychotherapy services. Participation in a supported housing program alongside her intensive mental health services has allowed her to live on her own and access supports when she relapses. She adopted a cat and reports a strong attachment and desire to nurture it—typical responses of individuals with less severe forms of mental illness who live with emotional support animals (see Chapter 3, "Roles of Animals With Individuals Who Have Mental Illness," for additional information about emotional support animals). Consistent with her motivation to provide a good environment for her cat, she cares for her apartment and practices routine self-care so that she will be healthy and available to care for her pet. Ms. K clearly experiences emotional benefits associated with attachment to a companion animal, including a sense of being loved and feeling less alone. Potential drawbacks of the situation include the need for her ACT team to care for the cat when Ms. K is hospitalized, which occurs periodically because of suicidal ideation.

This case highlights some of the positive influences of companion animals on mental health for people with SMI. It also illuminates the importance of ensuring that companion animals are not neglected when their owners are hospitalized. In this case, the ACT team took it on themselves to care for the cat. (Note, however, that some teams may not be able to take on this role, and in Ms. K's case no formal policy was provided for the welfare of the animal.) In support of animal welfare considerations, teams that provide intensive, in-home treatment in the context of supported housing programs may need to collaborate with local animal welfare agencies (Hoy-Gerlach et al. 2021) or to craft policies regarding who takes responsibility for the welfare of companion animals for patients.

Key Clinical Points

- Animal-assisted interventions (AAIs) and animal-assisted therapy (AAT) may be effective adjuncts to standard treatments for schizophrenia. Evidence suggests that AAIs for people with schizophrenia and related illnesses increase self-efficacy, coping, happiness, self-reported quality of life, and treatment adherence.

- Salutary effects of AAIs, AAT, and animal-assisted activities (AAAs) have been noted for positive symptoms of schizophrenia and, importantly, negative symptoms, which are notoriously intransigent.

- Equine-assisted therapy may have a unique role in treating long-term inpatients who struggle with aggressive behavior. Data do not currently support involving dogs in treating aggression in people with schizophrenia.

- Screening for dislike, fear, or aggression toward animals should be a requisite component of AAA, AAI, and AAT programs to protect animal, staff, and patient welfare. Animals involved in these interactions, especially residential or facility animals, should have a designated staff member to advocate for their welfare and well-being.

- Community-dwelling patients who wish to adopt an emotional support or companion animal should be made aware of the needs and behaviors of the pet and the financial commitment involved and should be able to provide long-term housing. Case managers should arrange to partner with local animal welfare agencies to provide for the animal's care if the owner becomes unable to do so.

- Care teams should be sensitive to psychiatric symptom exacerbation if patients experience grief over the death or loss of a companion animal and provide relevant supports.

- Robotic animals may be a useful substitute for individuals who are hospitalized, allergic to or fearful of animals, or unable to care for a pet of their own.

- Efforts should be made to provide formalized support for community-dwelling patients with companion animals to ensure the animals' welfare.

References

Abrahamson K, Cai Y, Richards E, et al: Perceptions of a hospital-based animal assisted intervention program: an exploratory study. Complement Ther Clin Pract 25:150–154, 2016 27863605

Adamou M: Community service models for schizophrenia: evidence-based implications and future directions. Psychiatry (Edgmont) 2(2):24–30, 2005 21179632

Artz B, Bitler Davis D: Green Care: a review of the benefits and potential of animal-assisted care farming globally and in rural America. Animals (Basel) 7(4):31, 2017 28406428

Bebbington P, Kuipers L: The predictive utility of expressed emotion in schizophrenia: an aggregate analysis. Psychol Med 24(3):707–718, 1994 7991753

Berget B, Braastad BO: Theoretical framework for animal assisted interventions: implications for practice. Ther Communities 29(3):323–337, 2008

Berget B, Braastad BO: Animal-assisted therapy with farm animals for persons with psychiatric disorders. Ann Ist Super Sanita 47(4):384–390, 2011 22194073

Berget B, Ekeberg O, Braastad BO: Animal-assisted therapy with farm animals for persons with psychiatric disorders: effects on self-efficacy, coping ability and quality of life, a randomized controlled trial. Clin Pract Epidemiol Ment Health 4(1):9, 2008 18405352

Brown AS, Meyer U: Maternal immune activation and neuropsychiatric illness: a translational research perspective. Am J Psychiatry 175(11):1073–1083, 2018 30220221

Calvo P, Fortuny JR, Guzmán S, et al: Animal assisted therapy (AAT) program as a useful adjunct to conventional psychosocial rehabilitation for patients with schizophrenia: results of a small-scale randomized controlled trial. Front Psychol 7:631, 2016 27199859

Chandler CK: An introduction to animal assisted therapy, in Animal Assisted Therapy in Counseling. New York, Routledge, 2012, pp 23–56

Chu C-I, Liu C-Y, Sun C-T, Lin J: The effect of animal-assisted activity on inpatients with schizophrenia. J Psychosoc Nurs Ment Health Serv 47(12):42–48, 2009 20000282

Corring D, Lundberg E, Rudnick A: Therapeutic horseback riding for ACT patients with schizophrenia. Community Ment Health J 49(1):121–126, 2013 22015959

Finnegan D, Onwumere J, Green C, et al: Negative communication in psychosis: understanding pathways to poorer patient outcomes. J Nerv Ment Dis 202(11):829–832, 2014 25357253

Gee NR, Rodriguez KE, Fine AH, Trammell JP: Dogs supporting human health and well-being: a biopsychosocial approach. Front Vet Sci 8:630465, 2021 33860004

Hall PL, Malpus Z: Pets as therapy: effects on social interaction in long-stay psychiatry. Br J Nurs 9(21):2220–2225, 2000 12271173

Hawkins EL, Hawkins RD, Dennis M, et al: Animal-assisted therapy for schizophrenia and related disorders: a systematic review. J Psychiatr Res 115:51–60, 2019 31108372

Hoy-Gerlach J, Vincent A, Scheuermann B, Ojha M: Exploring benefits of emotional support animals (ESAs): a longitudinal pilot study with adults with serious mental illness (SMI). Hum Anim Interact Bull 10(2):1–19, 2021

International Association of Human-Animal Interaction Organizations: The IAHAIO Definitions for Animal Assisted Intervention and Guidelines for Wellness of Animals Involved in AAI. Seattle, WA, IAHAIO, 2018. Available at: https://iahaio.org/best-practice/white-paper-on-animal-assisted-interventions. Accessed March 4, 2022.

Iwahashi K, Waga C, Ohta M: Questionnaire on animal-assisted therapy (AAT): the expectation for AAT as a day-care program for Japanese schizophrenic patients. Int J Psychiatry Clin Pract 11(4):291–293, 2007 24940729

Johnson JG, Cohen P, Dohrenwend BP, et al: A longitudinal investigation of social causation and social selection processes involved in the association between socioeconomic status and psychiatric disorders. J Abnorm Psychol 108(3):490–499, 1999 10466273

Jones PB, Rantakallio P, Hartikainen A-L, et al: Schizophrenia as a long-term outcome of pregnancy, delivery, and perinatal complications: a 28-year follow-up of the 1966 north Finland general population birth cohort. Am J Psychiatry 155(3):355–364, 1998 9501745

Jormfeldt H, Carlsson I-M: Equine-assisted therapeutic interventions among individuals diagnosed with schizophrenia: a systematic review. Issues Ment Health Nurs 39(8):647–656, 2018 29509053

Kessler RC, Birnbaum H, Demler O, et al: The prevalence and correlates of non-affective psychosis in the National Comorbidity Survey Replication (NCS-R). Biol Psychiatry 58(8):668–676, 2005 16023620

Kovács Z, Kis R, Rózsa S, Rózsa L: Animal-assisted therapy for middle-aged schizophrenic patients living in a social institution: a pilot study. Clin Rehabil 18(5):483–486, 2004 15293482

Lang UE, Jansen JB, Wertenauer F, et al: Reduced anxiety during dog assisted interviews in acute schizophrenic patients. Eur J Integr Med 2(3):123–127, 2010

Narita S, Ohtani N, Waga C, et al: A pet-type robot AIBO-assisted therapy as a day care program for chronic schizophrenia patients: a pilot study. Australas Med J 9(7):244–248, 2016

Nathans-Barel I, Feldman P, Berger B, et al: Animal-assisted therapy ameliorates anhedonia in schizophrenia patients: a controlled pilot study. Psychother Psychosom 74(1):31–35, 2005 15627854

Newbury JB, Arseneault L, Caspi A, et al: Association between genetic and socioenvironmental risk for schizophrenia during upbringing in a UK longitudinal cohort. Psychol Med 52(8):1527–1537, 2022 32972469

Nurenberg JR, Schleifer SJ, Shaffer TM, et al: Animal-assisted therapy with chronic psychiatric inpatients: equine-assisted psychotherapy and aggressive behavior. Psychiatr Serv 66(1):80–86, 2015 25269512

Olfson M, Gerhard T, Huang C, et al: Premature mortality among adults with schizophrenia in the United States. JAMA Psychiatry 72(12):1172–1181, 2015 26509694

Opler M, Charap J, Greig A, et al: Environmental risk factors and schizophrenia. Int J Ment Health 42(1):23–32, 2013

Palmer BA, Pankratz VS, Bostwick JM: The lifetime risk of suicide in schizophrenia: a reexamination. Arch Gen Psychiatry 62(3):247–253, 2005 15753237

Palumbo C, Volpe U, Matanov A, et al: Social networks of patients with psychosis: a systematic review. BMC Res Notes 8(1):560, 2015 26459046

Pugliese V, Bruni A, Carbone EA, et al: Maternal stress, prenatal medical illnesses and obstetric complications: risk factors for schizophrenia spectrum disorder, bipolar disorder and major depressive disorder. Psychiatry Res 271:23–30, 2019 30458317

Sahebalzamani M, Rezaei O, Moghadam LF: Animal-assisted therapy on happiness and life quality of chronic psychiatric patients living in psychiatric residential care homes: a randomized controlled study. BMC Psychiatry 20(1):575, 2020 33261578

Sallette L, King D, Cowton-Williams S, Mohan R: Patient and staff perceptions of animal-assisted therapy in psychiatric rehabilitation. BJPsych Open 7(S1):S216–S217, 2021

Seredova M, Maskova A, Mrstinova M, Volicer L: Effects of hippotherapy on well-being of patients with schizophrenia. Arch Neurosci 3(4):e39213, 2016

van de Leemput J, Hess JL, Glatt SJ, Tsuang MT: Genetics of schizophrenia: historical insights and prevailing evidence. Adv Genet 96:99–141, 2016 27968732

Wagner C, Lang UE, Hediger K: "There is a cat on our ward": inpatient and staff member attitudes toward and experiences with cats in a psychiatric ward. Int J Environ Res Public Health 16(17):3108, 2019 31461841

Wisdom JP, Saedi GA, Green CA: Another breed of "service" animals: STARS study findings about pet ownership and recovery from serious mental illness. Am J Orthopsychiatry 79(3):430–436, 2009 19839680

Wu EQ, Shi L, Birnbaum H, et al: Annual prevalence of diagnosed schizophrenia in the USA: a claims data analysis approach. Psychol Med 36(11):1535–1540, 2006 16907994

12

Companion Animals Assisting Patients in Hospice

Lisa D. Townsend, Ph.D., LCSW

I OUTLINE THE ROLE of companion and therapy animals in providing relief to patients undergoing hospice (end-of-life) care and their loved ones. I review research examining the effects of interacting with animals on outcomes such as anxiety, depression, and treatment receptiveness and highlight factors to consider when implementing an animal-assisted intervention (AAI) program in palliative settings. Formalization of human-animal interactions in the patient's care plan allows providers to link the visits to specific treatment goals and outcomes (International Association of Human-Animal Interaction Organizations 2018). In contrast, animal-assisted activities, such as unstructured therapy animal visits to a hospice facility, are not linked to specific patients' care plans. The chapter concludes with a case example of how a hospital-based dog/handler team helped a young woman cope with the death of her husband and a call for advocacy to elicit greater support for research on animal-assisted palliative care work.

Palliative care is a multidisciplinary specialty that provides holistic care for individuals who are facing illnesses associated with suffering, including physical pain, emotional distress, and spiritual difficulty (International Association for Hospice and Palliative Care 2019). Approximately 40 million people worldwide require palliative care each year

(World Health Organization 2020). Although palliative care focuses on alleviating suffering for a variety of illnesses and stages of disease, the human-animal interaction segment of this chapter covers end-of-life hospice care specifically.

Clinical Presentation and Longitudinal Time Course

A patient's health care provider can make hospice referrals when they determine that the patient has 6 months or less to live. Care focuses on the person's comfort and quality of life and is typically initiated when providers determine that further attempts to cure or stop the progression of illness will not succeed. Treatments provided during hospice care are comfort-based rather than curative. A team of individuals surrounds the patient during hospice care, including physicians, nurses, social workers, and clergy as needed. The patient can be served at home or in a hospital, nursing home, or dedicated hospice facility (National Institute of Aging 2021).

Overview of Existing Evidence-Based Treatments

Palliative medicine is a relatively new discipline, with formal board certification offered since 2008 (American Board of Internal Medicine 2021). Clinical care guidelines focus on holistic care for the patient, support for caregivers and family members, and treatments that range from pharmacotherapy for pain management to spiritual, psychological, and legal supports. Existing evidence shows promise for complementary approaches such as music therapy (Ahluwalia et al. 2018). Examinations of palliative treatments on intensive care units suggest that these interventions shorten length of stay and improve provider communication and consensus without increasing mortality (Aslakson et al. 2014). Patient- and family-centered decision-making represents one of seven key quality indicators for hospice care (Clarke et al. 2003).

Human-Animal Interactions and Mental Health Outcomes in Hospice Care

AAIs in hospice care can involve patients receiving visits from their own pets (pet visitation) or from therapy animals (therapy animal visits) who are approved to visit end-of-life care facilities. Research suggests that these visits are welcomed by staff, patients, and family members and are associated with psychological benefits and improved adherence to treatment.

Research indicates that even brief, one-time visits with a therapy dog reduce anxiety among patients in hospice care. Scagnetto et al. (2020) conducted a single-group design study of 44 patients at the end of life, measuring anxiety and depression outcomes. Participants received one 20-minute visit with a therapy dog. Anxiety was significantly decreased postintervention. Notably, however, anxiety reduction effects were significant only for current or past pet owners. This suggests a potential role of pet ownership in moderating outcomes of AAIs for palliative care patients, and further exploration is warranted.

Evaluations of longer-term therapy animal visitation interventions indicate that interacting with animals can decrease fear, despair, loneliness, and isolation for patients facing terminal illness. Muschel (1984) conducted a 10-week shelter animal hospice visitation program with 15 terminally ill oncology patients. Most of the patients reported benefits from the intervention, including being able to laugh and feeling warmth and closeness from holding an animal. Of the 3 patients who chose not to participate in the visits, 2 remained withdrawn and did not engage, and the third reported that although she had always loved animals, she was intentionally separating from relationships as she prepared to pass away. Data from studies like this one suggest that AAI visits are feasible and welcome for most patients in hospice care and that interactions with dogs can provide comfort and distraction for patients and their families.

Case study data uncover possible mechanisms by which visits with animals reduce emotional distress and physical symptoms for patients at the end of life. One such example is described by Quintal and Reis-Pina (2021), who outlined the benefits of pet visits for a 76-year-old woman with advanced colorectal cancer. Her treatment team facilitated weekly visits with her Yorkshire terrier, who was being cared for by her daughter. Providers noted that the patient required fewer rescue medications for pain and dyspnea on pet visit days than on non–pet visit days. The patient reported decreased anxiety and depression as well, observing that the hospital environment seemed more familiar when her dog was present. The hypothesized mechanism for the reductions in pain and dyspnea was relaxation, which is known to have salutary effects on physiological and psychological stress. Data from another case study that gathered observations from 19 palliative care patients also indicate that therapy dog visits may be associated with reductions in both pain and refusal of care (Engelman 2013).

Geisler (2004) provided clinical observations of hospice patients' reactions to visits from dogs in a hospital-based therapy dog program. Benefits shown by patients included a sense of caring for another life rather than being only the recipient of care; facilitating conversations between patients, family members, and staff; allowing patients to review positive aspects of their lives; and feeling close to another living being during a time of intense emotional isolation. The case study recommends gathering pet ownership history from hospice patients at program entry and incorporating therapy animal visits into patients' care plans.

AAIs can fulfill important elements of care plans, which are necessary in order for providers to receive reimbursement for hospice services. Medicare plan-of-care guidelines require documentation of individualized patient and family goals, services necessary for relieving symptoms of illness, and provision for the person's psychosocial and emotional needs (Center for Medicare Services 2021). Identifying whether patients can benefit from therapy animal visits or visitation by the patient's pet can be part of assessment and goal setting when an individual enters hospice care. The length and frequency of animal visits can be individualized according to patient and family preference and program capacity. In addition, volunteers are frequently vital elements of hospice care plans and can serve as important, cost-effective components of the patient's care team.

Animal-Assisted Intervention/Therapy Program Development and Implementation

Developing a well-run therapy animal program requires significant commitment, planning, knowledge, and buy-in from a variety of stakeholders. Giuliano et al. (1999) provide a template for initial animal-assisted intervention/therapy program development and implementation in a critical care setting, from writing an initial program manual to seeking feedback from stakeholders regarding visits. A summary of this process is found in Table 12–1.

Schmitz et al. (2017) provided insights into patient reactions to therapy dog visits in palliative care. The authors described the first year of a therapy dog visitation program in a university hospital–based palliative care unit (Schmitz et al. 2017) and offered a snapshot of what AAIs look like in hospice care contexts. The program was implemented with two dog-plus-handler teams who visited 52 patients and their family mem-

Table 12–1. Steps for animal-assisted intervention/therapy program development and implementation in critical care settings

Create program outline and guidelines.

Obtain buy-in from medical staff.

Develop safety protocols.

Formalize procedures and communicate them to stakeholders (e.g., how patients can request animal visits).

Prepare documentation.

Elicit feedback from patients, staff, and administrators.

bers over the course of a year. Most of the patients were in hospice care for terminal cancer. Visits lasted approximately 30 minutes on average; most patients received one visit, although most requested additional visits. During a typical visit, patients would pet and feed the dogs as well as engage them in tricks or obedience training. Some patients were able to walk outside with the handlers and their dogs. During these interactions, handlers conversed with patients about a variety of topics, which ranged from symptoms, death, and the process of dying to humorous anecdotes and the emotional connections humans have with animals.

Qualitative data were collected from the first year of program operations. Findings suggested that patients enjoyed physical contact with the dogs and that touching and petting the animals was a vital catalyst for benefits experienced by patients. Conversations ranged from lighthearted and humorous to serious and reflective. Some patients had greater motivation to engage in physical activity during the visits. Patients who were hesitant to engage with a dog shared feelings of sadness that they might become emotionally attached to the animal and then pass away, removing future opportunities to interact.

A small literature exists regarding the role of pet visitation in ameliorating distress for those in hospice care. These data are associational by necessity, given the impossibility of randomly assigning people to pet ownership. Results suggest that patients prefer to spend time with their pets at the end of life and that preparing for their pets' care following their passing represents a significant concern for them (Chur-Hansen et al. 2014). These findings indicate that there may be a role for pet visitation in palliative care as well as the need for staff to aid dying individuals so that their pets' well-being can be secured.

Systematic planning for pet and therapy dog visits during hospice care is important for ensuring that patients, caregivers, and health care providers have safe, enjoyable experiences and that animal welfare is maintained. Giuliano et al. (1999) provided a template for structured planning for these visits in critical care settings. They included a set of recommendations for both therapy and companion animal visits, with consideration for the contingencies that apply to each. Additionally, they emphasized the importance of involving relevant staff members in planning and administering a pet visitation program. Surveys assessing staff and patient attitudes toward involving animals in a day hospice program indicated generally positive attitudes toward their presence. Benefits endorsed by individuals involved in such programs included feeling relaxed, creating a homelike atmosphere, improving mood, and facilitating social interactions (Phear 1996).

Clinical and Animal Welfare Considerations

Palliative care environments may be associated with a variety of environmental stressors that affect staff, patients, and animals, including sounds from medical equipment and heightened emotions. A sound animal-assisted therapy program should be conceptualized thoughtfully, with a complete risk assessment being a priority, along with input from medical professionals, unit staff, volunteer handlers, and animal behavior and welfare professionals.

The Lincoln Education Assistance with Dogs (LEAD) Assessment Tool (Brelsford et al. 2020) serves as a current best practice standard for risk assessment and mitigation in animal-assisted activities, education, interventions, and therapy. The tool provides a framework for identifying potential risks to both human and animal participants that can be modified to account for unique environments, such as hospice care. In addition to mitigating risks to the humans, the tool emphasizes the importance of animal welfare and advocating on animals' behalf when they experience stress. The LEAD tool can facilitate conversations with medical staff prior to initiating animal-assisted hospice programs and form a foundation for identifying environmental characteristics that could affect visits and obtaining staff buy-in. The LEAD framework also delineates key staff members who will assume responsibility for specific risk mitigation tasks.

Once a program is established, ongoing success is contingent on consistent risk assessment and mitigation strategies, maintaining communication with relevant hospital personnel, assuring fidelity to animal welfare and infection prevention standards, and monitoring program

Table 12–2. Examples of best practices for hospital-based animal-assisted intervention programs

Animal welfare	Therapy animal evaluation and registration
	Annual and as-needed veterinary examinations
	Visit time limits
	Handler serving as designated advocate for animal welfare during visits
Patient welfare	Screening for allergies and fear of dogs
	Awareness of contact precautions and implications for animal visit
Volunteer handlers	Registration with hospital volunteer services department
	In-depth knowledge about their animal's stress signals and when to end a visit
Infection prevention	Animal grooming before visits
	Use of hand sanitizer before and after contact with animal
	Use of barrier between animal and hospital beds
Program improvement	Continuing education regarding animal behavior and the human-animal bond
	Ongoing program evaluation through research and quality assurance measures

functioning. Barker and Gee (2021) described a model canine-assisted intervention program and best practices for maintaining safety and program integrity. These considerations are summarized in Table 12–2.

Palliative care offers an opportunity to help provide for the well-being of patients' pets as well. Hospice programs may wish to address patients' concerns about what will happen to their pets after their death (Chur-Hansen et al. 2014) and provide resources for families to secure care for their loved ones' pets (see "Palliative Care Resources for Families" section at the end of this chapter). These resources can help to reassure dying individuals that their pets will be well cared for and decrease stress for loved ones who may have to find a suitable placement for the pet at some point in the process. Formalizing these concerns in a patient's plan of care may ease concerns about a pet's welfare, reduce stress, and improve emotional well-being.

Quality and Strength of Evidence for Animal-Assisted Interventions in Palliative Care

A recent systematic review of AAIs in oncology care highlights a fair degree of methodological consistency across studies, particularly in the involvement of dogs in the interventions, exclusion of high-risk patients, and infection prevention protocols (Holder et al. 2020). Common target outcomes included physical and psychological indicators. Overall, studies found significant beneficial effects on oxygen consumption outcomes and no significant effects on other physical parameters such as heart rate, blood pressure, and cortisol levels. Effects on psychological parameters were more robust, with studies indicating reduced anxiety, depression, hostility, and aggression as well as increased quality of life. Across studies, patients reported high levels of satisfaction with the AAIs and improved quality of life (Holder et al. 2020). A second systematic review replicated these findings, reporting significant improvements in depression among palliative care patients but no significant effects of AAIs on stress biomarkers (Diniz Pinto et al. 2021).

Studies of companion animal visits and more formal AAIs in hospice care have some methodological limitations (MacDonald and Barrett 2015), including small sample sizes, lack of randomization, and intervention heterogeneity. Few randomized controlled trials (RCTs) have been conducted in this area of medicine, and study populations vary along a wide range of characteristics, such as illness type and degree of ability to interact actively with the animals (Chur-Hansen et al. 2014). Overall, evidence suggests that hospice patients, families, and providers view AAIs as beneficial and desirable and that these programs are associated with palliative psychological and physical effects.

Some evidence suggests that AAIs may provide improvements in mood, anxiety, and pain (MacDonald and Barrett 2015). A review of studies in pediatric critical care suggested that AAIs are associated with improved mood, distraction from pain, and improved physiological parameters such as blood pressure and respiratory rate (DeCourcey et al. 2010). Recruitment for RCTs in palliative care is frequently beset with a variety of obstacles, which may partly explain the rarity of such studies. A recent study of older adults in critical care highlighted the complexities involved in successfully recruiting and completing data collection with this population. Branson et al. (2020) attempted to study a canine-assisted visit condition compared with treatment as usual for critically ill older adults. Although they successfully completed study procedures with 10 patients, a host of obstacles prevented the investigators from reaching their planned recruitment goal of 40 patients. Factors that prevented full recruitment included the severity of patients' illnesses, patients' inability to provide consent, and pain. Although this study was done in critical care, insights from the authors' experiences are highly relevant to investigators' ability to conduct RCTs in palliative care because of the high degree of overlap between the two populations. Specifically, illness severity, patient sedation, and pain likely serve as barriers to conducting RCTs in hospice care; the authors suggested obtaining consent from a legal proxy and using passive outcome measures as potential means for including more critically ill patients in RCTs of AAIs.

Areas for Future Research

Although conducting RCTs in hospice and critical care settings is difficult, the palliative care field could be advanced through the knowledge gained from such trials. Although single-group designs and qualitative or case studies provide valuable insights about how animal-assisted palliative care is perceived, they do not provide data on causal effects and the mechanisms by which these are achieved. The field would be well served by information about whether AAIs affect important outcomes for dying individuals and their families as well as the mechanisms by which they do so. If challenges related to the population or clinical context preclude RCT designs, well-characterized observational studies with multiple time points may provide a more feasible alternative (Vincent 2010).

The relationship of pet ownership to end-of-life issues represents another area in which scientific knowledge is sparse. We currently have little information about whether and how pet ownership moderates the effects of AAIs or how pet visitation programs might lessen the strain of dying on patients and their families. Given data suggesting that patients value their pets greatly and benefit from spending time with them at the end of life, the efficacy of pet visitation for people in hospice care needs greater exploration.

Case Example

Mr. M, a 35-year-old man with a wife and two young children, received a traumatic brain injury in an accident at work. Initially, his family and medical providers held out hope that he would show signs of recovery, but he slipped into a coma from which he never awakened. Mr. M's wife was faced with the difficult decision of discontinuing life support. While he lingered for several days with family members by his side, Mrs. M learned about a therapy dog visitation program that operated where he was hospitalized. She requested several visits after life support was discontinued, telling the staff that Mr. M loved dogs and would have loved to have seen his own dog one more time. A seasoned therapy dog team visited the couple during this time. The handler, Ms. L, had many years' experience in a hospital setting and listened while Mrs. M shared memories of Mr. M's relationship with their dog and the many fun adventures they had. The therapy dog, Merry, had an uncanny ability to sit quietly and lean into people who were suffering emotionally. Merry would often seek out people who were struggling the most, even if their struggle was not readily apparent to others. At Mrs. M's request, Merry stood next to Mr. M's bed, and his hand was placed on her head; this was meaningful to Mrs. M, who wanted him to have the chance to touch Merry in case he could sense her presence.

Ms. L and Merry were present during Mr. M's final moments and remained to comfort Mrs. M and other family members who had gathered at his bedside. Merry then sought out medical staff and sat next to the nurse who had provided most of Mr. M's care. His death proved to be especially difficult for providers because he and his family were so young and the accident so unexpected. The effusive gratitude the family and staff extended to Ms. L and Merry for their consistent presence during Mr. M's final days, and especially at the moment of his passing, highlights the ways in which the potential benefits of AAIs in a palliative care environment can extend beyond the patient.

Palliative Care Resources for Families

We recommend using patient- and family-centered care models for patients in palliative care as well as reinforcement-based training methods for therapy dogs and companion animals. The example resources that follow were reviewed for inclusion of patient-centered care and positive/reinforcement-based training for therapy dogs. We do not endorse aversive conditioning or punishment-based training methods for animals. The content of websites may change over time; therefore, we suggest reviewing resources before implementing them in patient care or animal training.

1FUR1 Foundation www.1fur1.org	Program available in Illinois, California, Michigan, Missouri, Florida, Tennessee, South Carolina, and North Carolina that provides animal-assisted activities and animal-assisted therapy in several types of facilities

911fosterpets https://911fosterpets.com	Online community that connects people to temporary homes and fostering for their pets
Best Friends https://bestfriends.org	Animal sanctuary in Utah that provides housing, fostering, and nationwide adoption services
Humane Rescue Alliance www.humanerescuealliance.org/ rehoming-resources	Rehoming resources and tips
Pet Partners https://petpartners.org/blog/ guest-post-reflections-on- therapy-animal-work-in-hospice	National therapy dog registration program with a mission to improve human health and well-being through the human-animal bond
Richmond SPCA https://richmondspca.org/what- we-do/programs-services/ surrender-your-pet	Organization that helps assist pet owners with free listings and may offer temporary housing
Ultimate Plus Hospice Pet Therapy and Rehoming Programs https://ultimateplushospice.com/ home-health-care-programs/pet- therapy-and-rehoming	Hospice center in Texas (Dallas–Fort Worth area) that provides pet therapy and assistance with rehoming patients' pets if needed

Key Clinical Points

- Existing studies suggest that animal-assisted interventions (AAIs) are associated with pain reduction, reduced feelings of social isolation, improvements in anxiety and depression, and greater cooperation with treatment among palliative care patients.

- Properly designed AAIs, whether they involve a patient's pet or a volunteer therapy dog team, can be incorporated into a patient's formal plan of care at minimal expense.

- A well-structured AAI program for a palliative care environment should adhere to best practices guidelines as described in the tables included in this chapter, with additional information available through referenced publications. A key component to such a program is advance buy-in from medical professionals.

- Assessing pet ownership and the potential role of pet visitation programs may be of potential benefit to palliative care patients and their families.

- Providing for their pets' care after their passing represents a significant concern for pet owners approaching the end of their lives. Strategies for addressing these concerns can provide significant relief for patients and their loved ones.

References

Ahluwalia SC, Chen C, Raaen L, et al: A systematic review in support of the National Consensus Project Clinical Practice Guidelines for Quality Palliative Care. J Pain Symptom Manage 56(6):831–870, 2018 30391049

American Board of Internal Medicine: Hospice and Palliative Medicine Policies. Philadelphia, PA, American Board of Internal Medicine, 2021. Available at: https://www.abim.org/certification/policies/internal-medicine-subspecialty-policies/hospice-palliative-medicine. Accessed August 28, 2021.

Aslakson R, Cheng J, Vollenweider D, et al: Evidence-based palliative care in the intensive care unit: a systematic review of interventions. J Palliat Med 17(2):219–235, 2014 24517300

Barker SB, Gee NR: Canine-assisted interventions in hospitals: best practices for maximizing human and canine safety. Front Vet Sci 8:615730, 2021 33869316

Branson S, Boss L, Hamlin S, Padhye NS: Animal-assisted activity in critically ill older adults: a randomized pilot and feasibility trial. Biol Res Nurs 22(3):412–417, 2020 32319313

Brelsford VL, Dimolareva M, Gee NR, Meints K: Best practice standards in animal-assisted interventions: how the LEAD risk assessment tool can help. Animals (Basel) 10(6):974, 2020 32503309

Center for Medicare Services: Creating an Effective Hospice Plan of Care. Baltimore, MD, Center for Medicare Services, 2021. Available at: https://www.cms.gov/files/document/creating-effective-hospice-plan-care.pdf. Accessed January 2, 2022.

Chur-Hansen A, Zambrano SC, Crawford GB: Furry and feathered family members—a critical review of their role in palliative care. Am J Hosp Palliat Care 31(6):672–677, 2014 23892336

Clarke EB, Curtis JR, Luce JM, et al: Quality indicators for end-of-life care in the intensive care unit. Crit Care Med 31(9):2255–2262, 2003 14501954

DeCourcey M, Russell AC, Keister KJ: Animal-assisted therapy: evaluation and implementation of a complementary therapy to improve the psychological and physiological health of critically ill patients. Dimens Crit Care Nurs 29(5):211–214, 2010 20703127

Diniz Pinto K, Vieira de Souza CT, Benamor Teixeira ML, Fragoso da Silveira Gouvêa MI: Animal assisted intervention for oncology and palliative care patients: a systematic review. Complement Ther Clin Pract 43:101347, 2021 33691267

Engelman SR: Palliative care and use of animal-assisted therapy. Omega (Westport) 67(1–2):63–67, 2013 23977780

Geisler AM: Companion animals in palliative care: stories from the bedside. Am J Hosp Palliat Care 21(4):285–288, 2004 15315191

Giuliano KK, Bloniasz E, Bell J: Implementation of a pet visitation program in critical care. Crit Care Nurse 19(3):43–50, 1999 10661091

Holder TRN, Gruen ME, Roberts DL, et al: A systematic literature review of animal-assisted interventions in oncology (part I): methods and results. Integr Cancer Ther 19:1534735420943278, 2020 32815410

International Association for Hospice and Palliative Care: Consensus-based definition of palliative care. Houston, TX, International Association for Hospice and Palliative Care, 2019. Available at: https://hospicecare.com/what-we-do/projects/consensus-based-definition-of-palliative-care. Accessed August 21, 2021.

International Association of Human-Animal Interaction Organizations: The IAHAIO Definitions for Animal Assisted Intervention and Guidelines for Wellness of Animals Involved in AAI. Seattle, WA, IAHAIO, 2018. Available at: https://iahaio.org/best-practice/white-paper-on-animal-assisted-interventions. Accessed April 16, 2021.

MacDonald JM, Barrett D: Companion animals and well-being in palliative care nursing: a literature review. J Clin Nurs 25(3–4):300–310, 2015 26522914

Muschel IJ: Pet therapy with terminal cancer patients. Soc Casework 65(8):451–458, 1984 10268446

National Institute of Aging: What are palliative care and hospice care? Bethesda, MD, National Institute of Aging, 2021. Available at: https://www.nia.nih.gov/health/what-are-palliative-care-and-hospice-care. Accessed December 31, 2021.

Phear DN: A study of animal companionship in a day hospice. Palliat Med 10(4):336–338, 1996 8931070

Quintal V, Reis-Pina P: Animal-assisted therapy in palliative care. Acta Med Port 34(10):690–692, 2021 32955417

Scagnetto F, Poles G, Guadagno C, et al: Animal-assisted intervention to improve end-of-life care: the moderating effect of gender and pet ownership on anxiety and depression. J Altern Complement Med 26(9):841–842, 2020 32924558

Schmitz A, Beermann M, MacKenzie CR, et al: Animal-assisted therapy at a university centre for palliative medicine: a qualitative content analysis of patient records. BMC Palliat Care 16(1):50–62, 2017 28969619

Vincent JL: We should abandon randomized controlled trials in the intensive care unit. Crit Care Med 38(10 Suppl):S534–S538, 2010 21164394

World Health Organization: Palliative care: key facts. Geneva, World Health Organization, 2020. Available at: https://www.who.int/news-room/fact-sheets/detail/palliative-care. Accessed August 21, 2021.

13

Companion Animals in the Treatment of Dementia and Aging-Related Concerns

Nancy R. Gee, Ph.D.
Jessica Bibbo, Ph.D.
Laura Dunn, M.D.

THE LITERATURE ON how companion animals may impact the lives of older adults tends to focus on one of two distinct perspectives on human aging: 1) aging as the single greatest risk factor for mortality (McCune and Promislow 2021) or 2) aging as an opportunity for improving health, well-being, and quality of life (Mueller et al. 2018). The first perspective focuses on illnesses, such as Alzheimer's disease, whose incidence increases with age, as well as aging-related decrements in functioning and quality of life, such as loss and loneliness. In contrast, the second perspective emphasizes the concept of "successful aging," which includes four key components: 1) avoiding disease and disability; 2) maintaining high-functioning physical, mental, and cognitive capacity; 3) active engagement; and 4) psychological adaptation (Kim and Park 2017). In this chapter, we consider the relevant science from both perspectives to establish an understanding of the ways that animals may alleviate or forestall disease, or improve health, well-being, and quality of life. We also present specific examples of incorporating animals into treatment plans for older adults.

Clinical Presentation, Prevalence, and Risk Factors

Aging-Related Concerns for Older Adults

Changes in functioning are unavoidable aspects of aging. However, these changes become concerns when they negatively affect an older adult's ability to navigate everyday life. These essential daily functions, known as *activities of daily living* (ADLs), are tasks that must be performed to care for oneself and remain independent (Edemekong et al. 2022). These tasks are sometimes grouped into two categories: 1) basic ADLs, those tasks that are essential to manage physical well-being (e.g., feeding, dressing, toileting), and 2) instrumental ADLs, those that require complex thinking and organizational skills required to maintain independence (e.g., shopping and meal preparation, managing finances, transportation). In this chapter, we simply use *ADLs* to denote all activities and tasks required to live independently.

Changes in physical, cognitive, or sensory functioning can all lead to decreased ability to perform ADLs (Crews and Campbell 2004; Edwards et al. 2020; Vaughan et al. 2016). Moreover, greater limitations in functioning increase the likelihood of experiencing social isolation (National Academies of Sciences, Engineering, and Medicine 2020). Prior to the coronavirus SARS-CoV-2 disease (COVID-19) pandemic, as many as 24% of community-dwelling older adults experienced social isolation (Cudjoe et al. 2020). The pandemic significantly exacerbated this underlying problem, which resulted in numerous deleterious downstream effects on the mental and physical well-being of older adults (MacLeod et al. 2021).

Depression in Older Adults

Depression can have many etiologies, including social isolation; loneliness; acute changes in health, such as a myocardial infarction or stroke; and chronic health conditions, such as cancer or pain, as well as socioeconomic and genetic causes (Fiske et al. 2009). Although less than 5% of older adults in the community live with major depressive disorder (Centers for Disease Control and Prevention 2021), this rate rises to more than 10% when an older adult is hospitalized or requires home health care. Depression is associated with a decline in cognitive functioning (Donovan et al. 2017) and mortality (Schulz et al. 2000), as well as presentations involving somatic complaints (e.g., insomnia, pain) or irritability (Fiske et al. 2009). Depression can be successfully treated in older adults, and doing so also may increase physical functioning (Callahan et al. 2005).

A systematic review of the literature found that depressive disorders were the most common risk factor for suicidal behavior in older adults (Beghi et al. 2021). In addition to depression, other risk factors for suicide in older adults include social isolation, perceived poor health, barriers to access to psychotropic medication, impaired sleep, previous suicide attempts, chronic diseases (e.g., cancer), and functional impairment (Fässberg et al. 2016). The lethality rate of attempted suicide increases with age and is higher in males than in females (Dombrovski et al. 2008). Although these statistics are alarming, interventions that promote a holistic view of health and well-being, including social connectedness, can have a positive effect on older adults at risk for suicide (Conwell 2014).

Dementia in Older Adults

Dementia is not a normal part of aging but rather an umbrella term for progressive diseases characterized by the deterioration of cognitive functioning and the ability to perform everyday activities (World Health Organization 2020). Dementia is one of the leading causes of disability among older adults worldwide (World Health Organization 2020), with an estimated 50 million people currently living with dementia and another 10 million new cases reported every year. Dementia has a broad range of effects—including psychological, physical, economic, and social—on affected individuals, their families and caregivers, and society as a whole.

Although many causes and forms of dementia have been identified, the most common type is Alzheimer's disease, which is estimated to represent 60%–70% of cases (Kim et al. 2021). Despite billions of dollars invested over decades, no consistent disease-modifying treatments are available for Alzheimer's disease. Given the relative failure of pharmacological strategies to halt or slow the progression of Alzheimer's disease and other dementias, nonpharmacological interventions and adjuncts to treatment are receiving considerable attention for their potential to slow cognitive decline and facilitate active engagement with the present. Animal-assisted interventions (AAIs) have been explored for their potential to improve emotional, social, and cognitive functions in older adults with dementia.

Potential for Companion Animals to Positively Affect the Lives of Older Adults

An accumulating body of evidence indicates that interacting with a companion animal can offer a range of potential benefits to older adults (Gee and Mueller 2019). Similarly, although based primarily on correlational data, evidence suggests that owning a companion animal also provides benefits. Such benefits include improvements in cardiac health and physiological responses to stress and increases in physical activity such as walking, as well as decreases in depression, anxiety, fear, agitation, and related behavior. Although the evidence is strongest with regard to physical health and depression, none of these health benefits has universally consistent research outcomes.

Scientific Evidence Base

Animals as Adjuncts in the Treatment of Aging-Related Concerns

Older Adults Living in the Community

Pet ownership is relatively common among the older adult population, with estimates ranging from 50% of adults older than 50 to 14% of those older than 65 (Mueller et al. 2018). However, companion animal ownership decreases dramatically with age. A recent study involving 378 participants in the Baltimore Longitudinal Study of Aging showed that the percentage of older adults who had pets was significantly lower across each advancing age category; 50.0% at 50–59 years, 35.3% at 60–69 years, 28.2% at 70–79 years, 14.4% at 80–89 years, and 0% at 90 years or older (Friedmann et al. 2020). Ironically, even though the aging population may have increasing difficulty in keeping their own companion animal, they may also be best poised to benefit from companion animal ownership.

In addition to potential health benefits, pets can provide a reason to get out of bed in the morning, a schedule to frame the day around, a companion to spend time with, and a positive topic of conversation with others. Pets also provide an important opportunity to nurture another and to give and receive affection. This bidirectional relationship can be particularly salient for those from historically marginalized populations, such as the lesbian, gay, bisexual, and transgender community (Muraco et al. 2018), and for any socially isolated individuals who do not have regular interaction with other people (Stanley et al. 2014). Pets tend to make people feel needed, valued, and loved, and studies indicate that they can fill Ainsworth's four roles of an attachment figure (Ainsworth 1989). Specifically, pets are 1) enjoyable, 2) comforting (Bonas et al. 2000), 3) missed when absent (Archer and Winchester 1994), and 4) sought in times of distress (Kurdek 2009).

The physical health benefits of companion animals to older adults tend to cluster around cardiac health, physical activity, and overall stress reduction. A recent systematic review (Gee and Mueller 2019) identified 26 studies that used standardized measures within cross-sectional, representative samples or longitudinal repeated measures. Findings indicated that a common outcome was the significant relationship between pet ownership and cardiac health. For example, pet presence was associated with lower blood pressure in older adults with hypertension (Friedmann et al. 2013); moreover, among 460 older adults recovering from a myocardial infarction, pet ownership was the only variable that significantly predicted survival (Friedmann et al. 2011). Several studies report that older adult dog owners engage in significantly more walking than do non–pet owners and that dog walking also includes some positive social outcomes resulting from increased community engagement (Gee and Mueller 2019).

The extant literature also has reported negative, mixed, or null results on cardiovascular outcomes. For example, among 242 patients admitted to a hospital for acute cardiac symptoms, pet owners (especially cat owners) had higher rates of mortality and readmission than did non–pet owners (Parker et al. 2010). It is also important to consider that overall health status may be a potential driver of the connection between pet ownership and positive cardiac health outcomes. Several studies have reported that poor health status is associated with a reduced likelihood of pet ownership (summarized in Gee and Mueller 2019). Even so, the American Heart Association reviewed the existing body of research and issued a scientific statement that pet ownership, particularly dog ownership, may play a causal role in reducing one's risk of cardiovascular disease (Levine et al. 2013).

The psychological health benefits of companion animals to older adults are less clear, and the mixed findings in the literature seem to indicate that the relationship, if any, is more complicated than can be easily assessed by a simple comparison of pet owners and nonowners. For example, an early study on recovery from bereavement in older adults reported that pet ownership and pet attachment were associated with less depression (Garrity et al. 1989). A more recent examination of the same topic reported that older adults facing a social loss without a pet had statistically greater increases in depressive symptoms than did those with a pet (Carr et al. 2020). Other studies have found no association between pet ownership and depression, and multiple studies have found that pet owners are more likely to be depressed than non–pet owners (Gee and Mueller 2019). Several possible explanations for these conflicting findings exist: 1) owning a pet may reduce or ameliorate depression; 2) depressed individuals may opt to acquire a pet as a means of self-help, leading to the population of pet owners having a higher proportion of people with depression than in the general population; 3) no causal relationship between pet ownership and depression exists; or 4) the relationship between pet ownership and depression is complicated and involves several known (e.g., physical activity and health) and unknown variables. Evidence indicates that the relationship between pet ownership and depression varies across groups of older adults, underscoring the complexity of this relationship. For example, in a population-based study of 12,093 older adults, female cat owners showed the highest levels of depression (Enmarker et al. 2015). This finding indicates that gender, age, and type of pet all may be critical factors in the relation between pet ownership and psychological health outcomes.

Although the empirical literature is mixed regarding the direct effect of pet ownership on health outcomes, older adults themselves consistently report strong, meaningful bonds with their pets. This bond, in conjunction with the responsibilities of pet ownership, can provide meaning and motivation for behaviors that support daily functioning (Obradović et al. 2020). For instance, people age 70 or older living with chronic pain reported that their pet played an important role in their daily health routines, including their management of mood, physical activity, and schedule (Janevic et al. 2020). Pets also may provide important support for older adults at risk for suicide. A qualitative study focused on the effect of pets on health uncovered evidence that the bidirectional support from and to a pet can be a protective factor against suicidal behavior (Young et al. 2020).

Older Adults in Residential Long-Term Care Facilities

A recent systematic review of 43 studies of AAIs involving dogs taking place in residential long-term care facilities highlighted several positive effects in that setting (Jain et al. 2020). The interventions carried out across studies varied widely but shared some common elements. For example, the most common dog breeds involved in the interactions were retrievers ($n=14$) and Labrador retrievers ($n=6$), informal dog visitation occurred most frequently for 30–90 minutes ($n=24$) once per week ($n=17$), with a pooled mean intervention period of 13.8 weeks, and in most studies the intervention group was compared with a control group that consisted of treatment as usual ($n=16$), social visits ($n=7$), or a robotic/plush toy ($n=4$). Nearly half of the studies reported no significant changes or differences ($n=18$, 46%) between groups. Of those that reported significant differences, the primary effects for older adults in residential long-term care facilities were improved social functioning ($n=10$), reduced depression ($n=6$), and reduced loneliness ($n=5$).

Animals as Adjuncts in the Treatment of Dementia

Continuing to engage in relationships and activities that were meaningful prior to the onset of dementia is associated with better quality of life postdiagnosis (Hennelly et al. 2021). Interactions with pets can provide people living with dementia a mechanism to connect with the world. A recent systematic review of 32 studies of AAIs in patients with dementia highlighted several positive effects (Yakimicki et al. 2019). Agitation or aggression was significantly reduced in 9 of 15 studies. Social interaction was significantly increased in 11 of 12 studies. Quality of life was increased in 3 of 4 studies, and mood had mixed results in 9 studies. Finally, activity level and nutritional intake were increased in 3 of 3 studies. In short, AAIs had a strong positive effect on social behavior, physical activity, and dietary intake, and a moderately positive effect on agitation or aggression and quality of life, in older adults with dementia.

Pets can have a significant effect on the lives of people living with dementia in the community, although pet ownership in this context has not been rigorously investigated. People living with Alzheimer's disease reported that pets continued to provide an important source of companionship (Shell 2015). Furthermore, pets did not judge individuals for behaviors that typically may be stigmatized during public interactions. However, changes in functioning may lead to changes in the relationship with a pet. A study of female spousal caregivers for husbands living with dementia reported both positive and negative changes in their husbands' relationship with the pet, whereas the changes in their own relationship to the pet were mostly positive (Connell et al. 2007). Negative changes in the husbands' relationship with their pet were related to less interaction with the pet (e.g., having no awareness of the pet, being less affectionate, spending less time), but positive changes centered on the pet playing a unique supportive role to the husband (e.g., promoting calm, providing a diversion or distraction, offering companionship). Pet dogs can continue to provide a necessary opportunity for physical activity for people living with mild to moderate dementia (Opdebeeck et al. 2021). The same study found that remaining actively involved in the care of a pet was essential to the pet's contribution to an individual's quality of life, underscoring the need to remain engaged in valued relationships and activities.

Quality and Strength of the Scientific Evidence Base

The scientific evidence described earlier in this chapter focuses on one of three perspectives—1) effects of owning a pet, 2) effects of contact with pets, or 3) AAIs—each of which includes complexities that influence research design elements (Friedmann and Gee 2019). Across all three perspectives there are challenges, including specifying health outcomes along with determining reliable and valid ways of measuring those outcomes; accessing participants who dislike, or who are allergic to, companion animals; and blinding participants and researchers to the presence of the animal in the study.

There are two major challenges to research on pet ownership: selection bias and defining pet ownership. Selection bias refers to the fact that most pet ownership research involves studying existing pet owners, who by definition have self-selected for ownership status (owner vs. nonowner) and for the type of pet they choose to own (e.g., dog, cat). Very few studies have assigned pet ownership status to the participants. One example of a study that did is a randomized controlled trial conducted in Korea in which community-dwelling older adults were randomly assigned to receive either health advice or health advice and five crickets in a cage (Ko et al. 2016). This approach to research is something of an anomaly when compared with the volume of research conducted on existing pet owners, in which an attempt is made, statistically, to eliminate all potential confounders, the efficacy of which is generally unknown. The end result is a requirement to discuss associations between variables rather than causation.

The second major challenge, defining pet ownership, concerns the frequent approach that researchers take to dividing their data into pet owners and non–pet owners for statistical analysis. Typically, participants are asked if they own a pet, and if they respond "yes," then the follow-up questions, if any, revolve around the number and type of each species of animal. This approach yields no information about the amount of interaction, the quality of involvement, or the emotional bond a given participant may have with the pet. An individual may report owning a pet because a dog resides in their home, but it is entirely possible that they are not the primary caregiver or that they dislike the pet and spend little if any time in the presence of the dog. To fully understand the effect of pet ownership, we must more fully describe and account for the variability associated with differing levels and types of interaction and quality of involvement.

Case Example

Ms. O, a 90-year-old woman, was diagnosed with depression by her primary care physician; she tried antidepressant medication, but after several months of continued weight loss and worsening mood and anxiety, Ms. O was eventually hospitalized. Her medication was adjusted, and she was evaluated as a potential candidate for electroconvulsive therapy (ECT). These treatments proved highly effective, and she continued these treatments as an outpatient.

Approximately 1 year after her discharge from the hospital, Ms. O moved to an assisted-living facility closer to her family. Away from her own home, she became increasingly depressed and anxious again and felt socially isolated despite the group setting. She expressed feeling nervous about meeting new people. Because she had enjoyed living with dogs in the past, her family asked her psychiatrist if a dog would make a good companion for Ms. O. The psychiatrist was concerned that the animal might be too much of a burden but felt that it was up to Ms. O. She agreed to give this a try, although she was not enthusiastic about the idea and expressed some anxiety about the new responsibility. After an initial adjustment period, Ms. O began to enjoy spending time with her dog, including taking him for several short walks every day. She made several friends while on these walks and began attending regular exercise classes. Her psychiatrist noted that her affect was brighter and less anxious and that she was now talking about her dog fondly and wanted to show her psychiatrist pictures of him. She continued her medications and outpatient ECT treatments without needing further adjustments for several years.

Implications for Clinical Practice

Pets of various species can facilitate increased social interactions among people. For the practicing clinician, an awareness of the potential benefits of pets, whether in the form of AAIs or as a topic of discussion, may help establish and build rapport with older adult clients. Current pet ownership will not be possible or desirable for all older adults, given that it can be both a source of support (as described earlier) and a source of stress (e.g., pet care, illness, housing, financial costs). Also, pets can influence medical care decisions; older adults may delay or avoid necessary medical care to prevent separation from the pet (Obradović et al. 2020).

However, asking older adults about any history of pets, their current pets (or other exposure to animals), and their feelings about interactions with pets/animals may help point toward potential avenues for improving the patient's physical and emotional well-being (Hodgson et al. 2017) and identify how pets fit into their support system. Hodgson et al. (2020) created six tools that clinicians can use to incorporate an animal into the care of a patient and that are all applicable for the treatment of mental illness.

Several examples of recommended skills are provided in Tables 13–1 and 13–2. First, ADLs might be improved or regularized through an activity that incorporates the patient's pet or a registered therapy animal (Table 13–1). Second, animals may help combat social isolation and loneliness, perhaps in ways that have not been previously identified for a given patient (Table 13–2). Providers should assess their patient's abilities, needs, and situation to determine which, if any, of these activities are likely to be useful and make recommendations accordingly. It is important to note that individuals who require assistance with their own ADLs are likely to require assistance with basic pet care (Bibbo and Proulx 2018).

Table 13–1. Example skill #1: carrying out activities of daily living

At home with pet dog	Animal-assisted activities	Animal-assisted therapy

Suggest that patients build a routine that includes their pet as a part of their schedule:
• Morning: toileting, feeding, general care such as brushing
• Midday: toileting, exercise, training, or play
• Evening: toileting, feeding, establishing a routine for bedtime
• Weekly: bathing, washing bedding
• Monthly: administering flea/tick/heartworm medication
	Invite registered therapy dog teams to interact with older adults in a nursing home. Activities may include
	• Greeting, petting, and interacting with the dogs
	• Socializing with the handlers and others present
	• Playing fetch with the dogs or signaling the dogs to perform tasks (e.g., sit, down, wave)
		Focus on specific skills to maintain or improve activities of daily living:
		• Fine motor movements:
		  – Remove and replace the dog's collar or tie a bow on the collar
		  – Brush the dog
		  – Put a scarf on the dog
		• Large motor movements:
		  – Leash walk the dog (use a second leash for safety)
		  – Throw a ball or toy for the dog

Table 13–2. Example skill #2: combating social isolation and loneliness

With their own pet dog	Activities with other animals	Animal-assisted activities—therapy dogs
Suggest that patients engage with other people and build their social networks through pet-related activities such as • Walking the dog in the patient's own neighborhood, at local parks, or at appropriate dog-friendly social events • Joining a local dog training club and taking classes to help the dog learn basic manners and social skills around other dogs • Getting involved in a dog activity, such as trick training or scent work	Propose additional ways of building social networks: • Volunteerism: Training their own dog to become a therapy dog and taking their dog to visit others • Volunteerism: Working at a local shelter to help dogs and cats to find homes • Offering to pet-sit or performing a dog-walking service for friends or neighbors	Consider ways of increasing communication and social connection: • Animal-assisted activities: 　– Encouraging discussion of previous pet ownership or interaction among the people present 　– Discussing ideas for future interactions or activities • Animal-assisted therapy: 　– Walking a dog using a dual leash through a facility to encourage interaction with others

Key Clinical Points

- Barriers to pet ownership may exist for older adults, but engaging in recollections about previous pets can be a helpful clinical tool.

- Patients can be asked about current and past pet experience. Addressing the topic of pet ownership can promote honest and productive communication with a client. Recognizing and acknowledging the bond with their pet may significantly affect important decisions, and transitions will allow for a more comprehensive understanding of a patient.

- Assuming that pet ownership is feasible for an older adult, caring for the pet can assist with maintenance of activities of daily living (suggestions are provided in Table 13–1).

- Companion animals can help older adults cope with social isolation and loneliness, either through activities associated with pet ownership or through unstructured animal-assisted activities or animal-assisted therapy (as described in Table 13–2).

References

Ainsworth MD: Attachments beyond infancy. Am Psychol 44(4):709–716, 1989 2729745

Archer J, Winchester G: Bereavement following death of a pet. Br J Psychol 85(Pt 2):259–271, 1994 8032709

Beghi M, Butera E, Cerri CG, et al: Suicidal behaviour in older age: a systematic review of risk factors associated to suicide attempts and completed suicides. Neurosci Biobehav Rev 127:193–211, 2021 33878336

Bibbo J, Proulx CM: The impact of a care recipient's pet on the instrumental caregiving experience. J Gerontol Soc Work 61(6):675–684, 2018 30001189

Bonas S, McNicholas J, Collis G: Pets in the network of family relationships: an empirical study, in Companion Animals and Us: Exploring the Relationships Between People and Pets. Edited by Podberscek AL, Paul ES, Serpell JA. Cambridge, UK, Cambridge University Press, 2000, pp 209–236

Callahan CM, Kroenke K, Counsell SR, et al: Treatment of depression improves physical functioning in older adults. J Am Geriatr Soc 53(3):367–373, 2005 15743276

Carr DC, Taylor MG, Gee NR, Sachs-Ericsson N: Psychological health benefits of companion animals following a social loss. Gerontologist 60(3):428–438, 2020 31504497

Centers for Disease Control and Prevention: Depression is not a normal part of growing older. Atlanta, GA, Centers for Disease Control and Prevention, 2021. Available at: https://www.cdc.gov/aging/depression/index.html. Accessed February 13, 2022.

Connell CM, Janevic MR, Solway E, McLaughlin SJ: Are pets a source of support or added burden for married couples facing dementia? J Appl Gerontol 26(5):472–485, 2007

Conwell Y: Suicide later in life: challenges and priorities for prevention. Am J Prev Med 47(3 Suppl 2):S244–S250, 2014 25145746

Crews JE, Campbell VA: Vision impairment and hearing loss among community-dwelling older Americans: implications for health and functioning. Am J Public Health 94(5):823–829, 2004 15117707

Cudjoe TKM, Roth DL, Szanton SL, et al: The epidemiology of social isolation: national health and aging trends study. J Gerontol B Psychol Sci Soc Sci 75(1):107–113, 2020 29590462

Dombrovski AY, Butters MA, Reynolds CF III, et al: Cognitive performance in suicidal depressed elderly: preliminary report. Am J Geriatr Psychiatry 16(2):109–115, 2008 18239196

Donovan NJ, Wu Q, Rentz DM, et al: Loneliness, depression and cognitive function in older U.S. adults. Int J Geriatr Psychiatry 32(5):564–573, 2017 27162047

Edemekong PF, Bomgaars DL, Sukumaran S, Levy SB: Activities of daily living, in StatPearls. Treasure Island, FL, StatPearls Publishing, 2022. Available at: http://www.ncbi.nlm.nih.gov/books/NBK470404. Accessed August 13, 2021.

Edwards RD, Brenowitz WD, Portacolone E, et al: Difficulty and help with activities of daily living among older adults living alone with cognitive impairment. Alzheimers Dement 16(8):1125–1133, 2020 32588985

Enmarker I, Hellzén O, Ekker K, Berg AG: Depression in older cat and dog owners: the Nord-Trøndelag Health Study (HUNT)-3. Aging Ment Health 19(4):347–352, 2015 24990174

Fässberg MM, Cheung G, Canetto SS, et al: A systematic review of physical illness, functional disability, and suicidal behaviour among older adults. Aging Ment Health 20(2):166–194, 2016 26381843

Fiske A, Wetherell JL, Gatz M: Depression in older adults. Annu Rev Clin Psychol 5:363–389, 2009 19327033

Friedmann E, Gee NR: Critical review of research methods used to consider the impact of human–animal interaction on older adults' health. Gerontologist 59(5):964–972, 2019 29668896

Friedmann E, Thomas SA, Son H: Pets, depression and long term survival in community living patients following myocardial infarction. Anthrozoos 24(3):273–285, 2011 21857770

Friedmann E, Thomas SA, Son H, et al: Pet's presence and owner's blood pressures during the daily lives of pet owners with pre- to mild hypertension. Anthrozoos 26(4):535–550, 2013

Friedmann E, Gee NR, Simonsick EM, et al: Pet ownership patterns and successful aging outcomes in community dwelling older adults. Front Vet Sci 7:293, 2020 32671105

Garrity TF, Stallones LF, Marx MB, Johnson TP: Pet ownership and attachment as supportive factors in the health of the elderly. Anthrozoos 3(1):35–44, 1989

Gee NR, Mueller MK: A systematic review of research on pet ownership and animal interactions among older adults. Anthrozoos 32(2):183–207, 2019

Hennelly N, Cooney A, Houghton C, O'Shea E: Personhood and dementia care: a qualitative evidence synthesis of the perspectives of people with dementia. Gerontologist 61(3):e85–e100, 2021 31854441

Hodgson K, Darling M, Freeman D, Monavvari A: Asking about pets enhances patient communication and care: a pilot study. Inquiry 54:46958017734030, 2017 28984509

Hodgson K, Darling M, Monavvari A, Freeman D: Patient education tools: using pets to empower patients' self-care—a pilot study. J Patient Exp 7(1):105–109, 2020 32128378

Jain B, Syed S, Hafford-Letchfield T, O'Farrell-Pearce S: Dog-assisted interventions and outcomes for older adults in residential long-term care facilities: a systematic review and meta-analysis. Int J Older People Nurs 15(3):e12320, 2020 32394594

Janevic MR, Shute V, Connell CM, et al: The role of pets in supporting cognitive-behavioral chronic pain self-management: perspectives of older adults. J Appl Gerontol 39(10):1088–1096, 2020 31215816

Kim S-H, Park S: A meta-analysis of the correlates of successful aging in older adults. Res Aging 39(5):657–677, 2017 27334287

Kim S, Nam Y, Ham MJ, et al: Neurological mechanisms of animal-assisted intervention in Alzheimer's disease: a hypothetical review. Front Aging Neurosci 13:682308, 2021 34335229

Ko HJ, Youn CH, Kim SH, Kim SY: Effect of pet insects on the psychological health of community-dwelling elderly people: a single-blinded, randomized, controlled trial. Gerontology 62(2):200–209, 2016 26383099

Kurdek LA: Pet dogs as attachment figures for adult owners. J Fam Psychol 23(4):439–446, 2009 19685978

Levine GN, Allen K, Braun LT, et al: Pet ownership and cardiovascular risk: a scientific statement from the American Heart Association. Circulation 127(23):2353–2363, 2013 23661721

MacLeod S, Tkatch R, Kraemer S, et al: COVID-19 era social isolation among older adults. Geriatrics (Basel) 6(2):52, 2021 34069953

McCune S, Promislow D: Healthy, active aging for people and dogs. Front Vet Sci 8:655191, 2021 34164450

Mueller MK, Gee NR, Bures RM: Human-animal interaction as a social deter-minant of health: descriptive findings from the health and retirement study. BMC Public Health 18(1):305, 2018 29519232

Muraco A, Putney J, Shiu C, Fredriksen-Goldsen KI: Lifesaving in every way: the role of companion animals in the lives of older lesbian, gay, bisexual, and transgender adults age 50 and over. Res Aging 40(9):859–882, 2018 29357737

National Academies of Sciences, Engineering, and Medicine: Social Isolation and Loneliness in Older Adults: Opportunities for the Health Care System. Washington, DC, National Academies Press, 2020

Obradović N, Lagueux É, Michaud F, Provencher V: Pros and cons of pet own-ership in sustaining independence in community-dwelling older adults: a scoping review. Ageing Soc 40(9):2061–2076, 2020

Opdebeeck C, Katsaris MA, Martyr A, et al: What are the benefits of pet owner-ship and care among people with mild-to-moderate dementia? Findings from the IDEAL programme. J Appl Gerontol 40(11):1559–1567, 2021 33025847

Parker GB, Gayed A, Owen CA, et al: Survival following an acute coronary syn-drome: a pet theory put to the test. Acta Psychiatr Scand 121(1):65–70, 2010 19522884

Schulz R, Beach SR, Ives DG, et al: Association between depression and mortal-ity in older adults: the Cardiovascular Health Study. Arch Intern Med 160(12):1761–1768, 2000 10871968

Shell L: The picture of happiness in Alzheimer's disease: living a life congruent with personal values. Geriatr Nurs 36(2 Suppl):S26–S32, 2015 25771956

Stanley IH, Conwell Y, Bowen C, Van Orden KA: Pet ownership may attenuate loneliness among older adult primary care patients who live alone. Aging Ment Health 18(3):394–399, 2014 24047314

Vaughan L, Leng X, La Monte MJ, et al: Functional independence in late-life: maintaining physical functioning in older adulthood predicts daily life func-tion after age 80. J Gerontol A Biol Sci Med Sci 71(Suppl 1):S79–S86, 2016 26858328

World Health Organization: Dementia. Geneva, Switzerland, World Health Or-ganization, 2020. Available at: https://www.who.int/news-room/fact-sheets/detail/dementia. Accessed February 13, 2022.

Yakimicki ML, Edwards NE, Richards E, Beck AM: Animal-assisted interven-tion and dementia: a systematic review. Clin Nurs Res 28(1):9–29, 2019 29441797

Young J, Bowen-Salter H, O'Dwyer L, et al: A qualitative analysis of pets as sui-cide protection for older people. Anthrozoos 33(2):191–205, 2020

14

Animal-Assisted Interventions for Improving the Mental Health and Academic Performance of University Students

Patricia Pendry, Ph.D.
Aubrey L. Milatz, M.S.
Alexa M. Carr, Ph.D.
Jaymie L. Vandagriff, Ph.D.

THE USE OF animal-assisted interventions (AAIs)—the practice of including animals in goal-directed interventions designed to prevent or treat physical or mental illness—has been increasing. Whereas some AAIs focus on treating psychiatric disorders through therapy, others incorporate animals as an avenue for *preventing* the development of psychopathology by alleviating symptoms associated with their development or strengthening factors associated with resilience during times of risk. In this chapter, we focus on an example of a prevention-oriented AAI approach—animal-assisted activities (AAAs). Commonly implemented by volunteers or paraprofessionals without therapeutic qualifications, AAAs lack a formal therapeutic approach but incorporate animals into programmatic interventions to improve individuals' quality of life and well-being by reducing stress or distress, providing social support, increasing motivation, creating a sense of community, and facilitating social interactions, as well as facilitating behavior change or the acquisition of new skills (International Association of Human-Animal Interaction Organizations 2018). We focus especially on university-based AAAs, a setting and population that have received tremendous attention from researchers, practitioners, and the public in response to what has been referred to as a "college student mental health crisis" facing postsecondary students worldwide (Henriques 2018).

Characteristics of University-Based Animal-Assisted Activities

University-based AAAs exist in a wide variety of forms. Planned and goal-oriented, most of these programs are animal visitation programs (AVPs) that arrange for animal/handler teams to visit a program site to facilitate informal interactions for as little as 10 minutes and up to several hours (Haggerty and Mueller 2017), often in the week leading up to students' examinations. Most AVPs conducted on university campuses feature dogs; however, the inclusion of cats and other animals is not unusual. In fact, in a geographically representative survey of university-based AVPs, Haggerty and Mueller (2017) reported that 86% of sampled programs featured dogs only; 5% featured cats and dogs; and 10% involved dogs, cats, and other species, including rabbits, baby goats, and alpacas. Because most AVPs are intended to provide access to numerous students in a relatively short time, they tend to involve supervised interactions in small group settings rather than one-on-one interactions. As the popularity of AVPs has grown and implementation has become widespread, a trend is emerging, with universities and colleges expanding the type and range of activities to include more structured, regular, and programmatic AAAs. These include regular drop-in programs (Binfet et al. 2018; Carr and Pendry 2022), workshops involving varying levels of psychoeducational content and human-animal interaction (HAI) with registered therapy canines (Pendry et al. 2020, 2021), and visitation programs in dorms and student organizations. Altogether, university-based AAAs are appealing to university administrators because they enjoy tremendous positive public perception and require less training and expertise than traditional therapies, allowing for low-cost implementation by volunteer organizations, which increases access to a greater and wider range of populations.

In the next section, we focus on the rationale for the increased popularity of, demand for, and implementation of universal and targeted campus-based AAIs and their most common purpose—alleviating student stress to prevent or modulate the development of stress-related disorders and associated academic failure. In subsequent sections, we examine implementation and evaluation approaches applied to campus-based AAIs, while emphasizing AVPs aimed at alleviating stress to mitigate the development of mental health disorders and academic failure in at-risk students. In addition to providing examples of various approaches to identify at-risk students, we present empirical evidence linking these approaches to results of efficacy trials featuring a range of programs and outcomes. Throughout, we discuss the strengths and limitations of the approaches used to identify at-risk populations. We close by reflecting on implementation and evaluation of campus-based AAIs within a context of increasing demand, limited capacity, policy-guided exceptions, and mixed evidence on sound practice.

The University Student Mental Health Crisis

The demand for campus-based AAIs is a response to university administrators' awareness of high rates of students' mental health problems and universities' limited capacity to provide services to address them. Even before the coronavirus SARS-CoV-2 disease (COVID-19) pandemic, 66.4% of students reported feeling "overwhelming anxiety," 46.2% felt "so depressed that it was difficult to function," and 14.4% seriously considered suicide (American College Health Association 2020). Moreover, academic stress played a huge role in creating elevated levels of stress; for example, more than half (52.7%) of the students reported that academic responsibilities were "traumatic or difficult to handle," 85% reported feeling exhausted (not from physical activity), and 88% felt overwhelmed by all they had to do (American College Health Association 2019). Unfortunately, the emergence of COVID-19 and consequences of the pandemic (e.g., closing of educational institutions, distance learning, social isolation) have further aggravated already serious mental health problems (Eisenberg and Lipson 2019; Lipson et al. 2019; Son et al. 2020). The Healthy Minds Network and American College Health Association

(2020) reported increased rates of students' depression (from 35.7% in fall 2019 to 40.9% in spring 2020), stable yet high rates of anxiety (31% at both time points), and a decrease in students' feelings of flourishing from 38.1% to 36.6%. Moreover, students reported increased rates of academic impairment due to anxiety (from 27.8% in 2019 to 31.1% in 2020) and depression (from 22.1% to 24.4% in that same time period). Finally, a whopping 81.8% of surveyed undergraduates reported an overall moderate or high level of stress within the past 12 months (Healthy Minds Network and American College Health Association 2020).

Risk Factors

In addition to the growing prevalence of perceived stress and symptoms of mental illness, reports indicate that individual risk factors increase the likelihood of perceiving high levels of stress and developing mental disorders. For example, there is a significant gap in the prevalence of symptoms and disorders by gender, with significantly higher rates for cis women than for cis men. Depression diagnoses were reported by 25.3% of cis women and 14.1% of cis men; 32.7% of women and 15.4% of men reported an anxiety diagnosis; 7.3% of women and 2.9% of men reported a diagnosis of PTSD; and 85.7% of women and 70.7% of men rated their overall level of stress experienced in the past 12 months as "moderate" or "high" (American College Health Association 2021). In addition, mental illness was particularly prevalent among the students who identified as transgender or gender nonconforming; 50.9% of these students reported a depression diagnosis, 54.9% reported an anxiety diagnosis, 18.9% reported a diagnosis of PTSD, and 89.5% reported moderate to high overall levels of stress within the last 12 months (American College Health Association 2021). Furthermore, students belonging to racial /ethnic minority groups may experience additional stress, anxiety, and depression related to discrimination and institutional racism (Greer and Cavalhieri 2019). These data clearly suggest that although the prevalence of stress-related disorders is high, with these disorders affecting one out of four students, students who are women, transgender, gender nonconforming, and of color are particularly vulnerable.

Overwhelming Demand on and Limited Capacity of University-Based Mental Health Centers

Although the links between stress exposure and psychopathology are complex, it is not surprising that universities have experienced an increase in demand for and use of interventions providing stress relief and counseling services (Lipson et al. 2019). Although university-based mental health centers are trying to respond accordingly, they face overwhelming demand and limited capacity. Data from 93 institutions show that the growth in on-campus counseling center appointments from 2008 to 2015 (38.4%) was more than seven times the growth in institutional enrollment (5.6%) for that period (Center for Collegiate Mental Health 2016). Many of these appointments reflect response-to-crisis situations rather than ongoing services; the proportion of rapid-access hours per client has increased by 28% over the past 6 years, whereas routine hours per client have decreased by 7.6% (Center for Collegiate Mental Health 2016). In fact, despite reporting elevated levels of stress and symptoms of mental illness, only 22.3% of students reported ever receiving psychological or mental health services from their university's counseling or health services (Center for Collegiate Mental Health 2016). These numbers fall short of the proportion of students who express interest in receiving information from their university: 72.9% of students expressed interest in stress reduction, 62.1% were interested in information on depression and anxiety, 54.8% expressed interest in suicide prevention, 67.7% expressed interest in information on helping others in distress, and 63.9% expressed interest in information on sleep difficulties. Interestingly, although students are eager to receive traditional counseling services, students' requests for campus-based AAIs have also increased, including requests for permission to reside with companion animals, a separate yet important aspect of campus-based AAIs that is discussed later (see section "Considering Companion Animals"). Given the tremendous need for and interest in interventions providing stress relief, the popularity of animal-assisted approaches, and the limited capacity to scale up animal-assisted programs while safeguarding animal well-being, our ability to identify and reach out to individuals most in need, or most likely to benefit from AAIs, has become paramount.

Identifying At-Risk Students in the Context of Campus-Based Animal-Assisted Interventions

As noted in the introduction to this chapter, we take a prevention science approach toward identifying participants most in need or most likely to benefit from AAIs. Prevention science is an interdisciplinary field that applies basic research about individuals, families, and communities to the development, evaluation, and dissemination of evidence-based programs, practices, and policies to promote physical, social, and psychological well-being. Within this approach, AAIs—and AVPs and AAAs in particular—are most often referred to as stress prevention programs whose approach varies depending on their closely related aims. Defined as "levels of prevention," AAIs may be conceptualized as a *universal* prevention that aims to prevent problems before they happen; a *selected* prevention that focuses on preventing a problem among a group of individuals identified as particularly at risk for the problem; or an *indicated* prevention that centers on preventing significant problems for a group of individuals already showing some indication that they have early stages of the problem (National Academies of Sciences, Engineering, and Medicine 2019). These definitions are conceptually similar to those used in the medical professions that categorize "levels of disease prevention" as primary, secondary, and tertiary prevention. Although AAIs can serve the goals associated with each of these levels of prevention, it is essential to consider the tools needed to successfully select the intended participants across these levels.

Various documented approaches are used to identify and consider at-risk students for AAI participation and to assess AAI effects on student outcomes of interest. Which approaches are most efficient or effective depends on the level of the intervention (e.g., universal, selected, indicated), type of implementation goals and strategy (e.g., walk-in or previous registration), stated research questions and hypotheses in cases when research and evaluation efforts are conducted (e.g., examination of risk status as moderating treatment effects), outcomes of interest (e.g., statelike or traitlike symptoms of disorders; physiological, behavioral, or cognitive functioning), and assessment tools (e.g., survey, diagnostic assessment, observed behavior). In the following section, we present examples of approaches that have been successfully used to identify and select students at various levels of risk, as well as assess differential treatment effects of AVPs and AAAs on outcomes of interest by risk status.

Selected Prevention Approach

Given the recent results of the American College Health Association (2021) report, one selected prevention approach is to identify at-risk students by drawing on shared demographic data collected by university registrars or by asking students to self-report demographic characteristics on an AAI registration/application form designed for the purpose. To avoid making students feel that they are being profiled, administrators can include questions about participants' characteristics not associated with risk status, such as their history of animal ownership, or breed and size preferences. It is important to consider using contemporary, diverse terms to describe gender; transgender status; use of preferred pronouns; and sex assigned at birth in cases in which the role or effect of AAIs on biological variables is explored. In addition, approaches that identify a diverse and inclusive set of indicators capturing race, ethnicity, and gender identity status are recommended. With these indicators, populations at risk for the development of stress-related disorders and academic failure can be identified, approached, and invited for participation accordingly.

Another selected prevention approach assesses student risk status beyond demographic indexes. This approach features a self-report screening tool embedded in a demographic survey aimed at identifying risk factors associated with the development of mental disorders or academic failure. Completing an internally developed screening survey, participants indicate whether they "have ever been declared academically deficient" and, if so, whether that status is current or whether they have been reinstated. They also indicate whether they "have ever been diagnosed with a mental health condition or disorder" and provide the diagnosis and date. Participants next indicate whether they "have ever seriously considered suicide or thought about harming themselves in any way" and indicate whether these thoughts occurred within the past month, semester, year, or prior. Last, participants check whether they "have ever received learning accommodations" and, if so, whether the provision occurs currently, within the past year, or prior. Risk of academic failure and mental disorder is operationalized by the *presence or history of risk* (0, 1) or a *cumulative history of risk* variable on a continuous scale (ranging from 0 to 4). These indicators are helpful for providing priority access during registration or indicated recruitment into AAI programs.

These specific risk factors were chosen because they are commonly used by university administrators and agencies to identify students eligible and suitable for referral and follow-up services. Students who indicate that they have experienced a diagnosed mental health condition or considered suicide or self-harm are eligible for referral to campus counseling and psychological services, where appropriate mental health practitioners can conduct diagnostic assessments. In addition, academically deficient students whose semester or cumulative grade point average dropped below 2.0 are required as part of their reinstatement process to participate in programs offered through student support services or campus health services providing counseling or health promotion. Similarly, the university provides students with learning disabilities options to apply for reasonable accommodations through the university's access center. Using a set of shared indicators can provide the benefits of streamlining and coordinating risk assessments while reducing burden on students and providing more efficient use of referral sourcing. Although this method provides practitioners little information about students' current level and nature of symptomatology, it provides useful screening information for referral to diagnostic assessments or personalized intervention.

Empirical Implications of a Selected Approach Assessing Risk and Treatment Effects

Empirical evidence suggests that a selected approach yields meaningful information for distinguishing treatment effects of AAI in university settings. Pendry et al. (2021) used this approach to oversample at-risk students and to examine whether effects of a 4-week AAI program on executive functioning varied for typical and at-risk college students. This outcome was of interest because executive functioning informs cognitive skills that have implications for academic functioning, such as paying attention, organizing, planning, and prioritizing; starting tasks and staying focused on them to completion; understanding different points of view; regulating emotions; and self-monitoring. In addition, evidence suggests that executive functioning is linked to mental health outcomes, including depression (Snyder 2013) and anxiety (Snyder et al. 2014), and indexes of social, cognitive, and psychological development as well as ADHD in college students (Jarrett 2016).

After screening, Pendry et al. (2021) used an experimental design comparing effects of risk status and three different combinations of HAI and evidence-based academic stress management (ASM) content over a 12-week assessment period. Conditions varied by the amount of HAI and featured 100% HAI, 100% ASM, or an equal combination of both (50% HAI and 50% ASM). Results immediately following the intervention showed significant improvements in global executive functioning and metacognition, achieved particularly for at-risk students who exclusively interacted with therapy dogs compared with at-risk students who received evidence-based ASM content or a combination of both. Moreover, the effects remained 6 weeks after program completion.

The observed improvements in executive functioning indicate that the amount of exposure to HAI embedded in an AAI is of paramount importance depending on the target population and their risk status. Although this study did not test mediating mechanisms potentially underlying the effects of HAI on executive functioning, the consistent effects of exclusive HAI exposure on executive functioning in at-risk students could be attributed to the fact that the interventions featuring HAI distracted these students from potential negative stressful thoughts, whereas attention to stress management strategies may have increased those thoughts. In fact, AAIs are thought to provide students with a novel, exciting, and enjoyable experience (Jau and Hodgson 2018), which may foster opportunities for momentary reprieves from negative thoughts related to mood disorders (Reinecke 2006), thus contributing to a calm, relaxed state, which is known to enhance executive functioning, especially in students with higher levels of risk. Also, the relaxed, calm state may have supported the development of other adaptive behaviors enhancing executive functioning skills, such as problem-solving, decision-making, and creative and critical thinking (Sahu and Gupta 2013), which we know were significantly lower at baseline in at-risk students. Most important, the result implies that a simple method of identifying at-risk students through examining their responses to four statements may, in future investigations and implementation efforts, be used to identify students most likely to benefit from interventions that emphasize HAI compared with traditional stress prevention efforts.

Indicated Prevention: Identifying Indicators of Stress-Related Psychopathology

To meet indicated prevention goals, researchers and practitioners can conduct comprehensive assessments to better understand the nature and level of participants' potential vulnerabilities and existing symptoms. Self-report measures can serve as risk indicators for developing mood and anxiety disorders, including assessments of anxiety (Beck Anxiety Inventory; Beck and Steer 1993), depression (Beck Depression Inventory; Beck et al. 1996), worry (Penn State Worry Questionnaire; Meyer et al. 1990), and perceptions of stress exposure (Perceived Stress Scale–10; Cohen 1994). Based on these self-report measures, a risk indicator (i.e., low or high) for each participant on each measure can be created from which a composite general mood risk indicator can be derived. One important logistical and ethical consideration is the need to share the results with participants and indicate that they should seek diagnostic assessment by a mental health professional because indicators suggest the presence of clinical levels of disorder. This communication needs to be conducted by a person with appropriate training and should be accompanied by confidential written communication indicating the presence of clinical levels, along with referral information and resources. These risk indicators can be used to provide priority access during registration or active recruitment into the AVP or AAA program. In addition, they are useful for conducting causal and pathway analyses within the context of a moderation model during efficacy trials.

Although this approach is more comprehensive than the selective approach, it increases the length of assessments for participants and requires expertise and resources to translate assessment data into meaningful indicators, which may prohibit the use of this approach for the purpose of immediate, targeted, personalized intervention in a fast-paced AVP environment. If the use of such assessments is feasible, they should be conducted within a reasonable time frame before the beginning of the intervention so that data can be ascertained, interpreted, and considered.

Empirical Implications of Using Mood and Perceived Stress as a Risk Indicator

Pendry et al. (2020) examined whether students' general mood risk, assessed as just described, moderated the effect of incorporating HAI into an evidence-based stress prevention program on students' studying and learning strategies. The results showed that interacting with therapy dogs and their handlers, either with or without exposure to formalized stress reduction content, improved behavioral aspects of academic success for university students classified as being at high risk based on the presence of higher-than-average stress-related mood symptoms, including depression, anxiety, perceived stress, and worry.

While the use of mood risk status based on combined self-reported assessments of depression, anxiety, worry, and perceived stress has yielded meaningful differences in students' behavioral improvements based on risk status, consideration of only one of these mood indicators has also shown differentiation of effects, albeit on different outcomes. Pendry et al. (2019) examined whether clinical levels of depression—as indicated by self-reported assessment of depressive symptoms only—moderated the effect of an AVP on university students' momentary emotional states (e.g., feeling content, anxious, irritable, and depressed) in response to varying conditions commonly experienced during college

AVPs. Findings showed that 10 minutes of hands-on HAI with shelter dogs and cats reduced negative emotional states (e.g., anxiety, irritability, depression) in participants reporting clinical levels of depression. Similarly, they found significant main effects on physiological stress relief as indicated by lower cortisol levels in depressed and nondepressed participants (Pendry and Vandagriff 2019). Interestingly, in a different study, Pendry et al. (2019) found that observing other students' pet cats and dogs while waiting in line—but not touching the animals themselves—offered some benefits to participants, *except* for clinically depressed students, who showed significantly higher levels of irritability, depression, and anxiety compared with those without clinical levels of depression in response to waiting in line. Given the significant interaction effects for waiting in line while observing others, these findings suggest that it is important to consider the conditions leading up to program participation, particularly for students experiencing clinical levels of depression, to prevent inadvertently increasing negative emotions in already depressed students. These results are relevant for those implementing AVPs, who must consider risk factors that may inadvertently negatively influence the experience of program participants, such as logistical challenges presented by discrepancies between defined program capacity (e.g., number of available animals and handlers) and greater-than-expected program uptake (e.g., long lines and overcrowding).

Assessing Pet-Related Separation Anxiety as a Risk Factor During the Transition to University

This chapter has focused on universities' efforts to enhance at-risk students' access to AAIs based on demographic characteristics, mental health symptoms, and academic performance. Little attention has been given to risk factors associated with the transition to university itself. One such phenomenon is animal-based separation anxiety among incoming university students, which occurs in response to leaving one's childhood pet behind. Pet-related separation anxiety has been measured by adapting the DSM-5 Severity Measure for Separation Anxiety Disorder, a 10-item measure that assesses the severity of symptoms of separation anxiety disorder in individuals age 18 years or older (Craske et al. 2013). Individuals rate the severity of the thoughts, feelings, and behaviors they may have experienced over the past 7 days, including "felt anxious, worried, or nervous about being separated [from my pet]," "felt tense muscles, felt on edge or restless, or had trouble relaxing or trouble sleeping when separated [from my pet]." Items are scored on a 5-point scale, with total scores ranging from 0 to 40. Higher scores indicate greater severity of separation anxiety. Scores can be categorized by symptom severity, ranging from none=0, mild=1, moderate=2, severe=3, and extreme=4. Using this measure (Cronbach α=0.86), Carr and Pendry (2022) showed that three of four students from a randomly selected sample of first-year students (n=145) reported mild or greater symptoms of pet-related separation anxiety in their first week on campus, with one in four reporting moderate or severe symptoms, which were positively associated with students' history of anxiety and self-harm. Whether students with pet-related separation anxiety benefit from AAIs is currently unknown but warrants examination because there is anecdotal evidence of students describing the loss of their pet as a loss of a coping resource against stress.

Considering Companion Animals

In addition to identifying who may benefit from exposure to "other people's animals," we should consider policies that grant students access to their own animals, including service animals, emotional support animals (ESAs), and pets. This topic was discussed in Chapter 3 ("Roles of Animals With Individuals Who Have Mental Illness"), but here we focus exclusively on issues related to university students. To understand the context in which university policies regarding companion animals are shaped, we refer to federal policies from which they stem: the Americans With Disabilities Act (ADA; 1990) and the Fair Housing Act (FHA; 1988). The ADA was created "to provide a clear and comprehensive national mandate for the elimination of discrimination against individuals with disabilities." The purpose of the FHA is to prevent property owners and housing associations from denying people housing based solely on the presence of a disability. It also requires property owners and housing associations to make reasonable accommodations for disabled tenants so that they can enjoy their dwelling to the same extent as nondisabled individuals.

There are three categories of companion animals: service animals, ESAs, and pets. Legal definitions were set forth by the ADA and FHA concerning "service animals," also referred to as "assistance animals"; under the ADA, service animals are legally defined as "any dog [or miniature horse] that is individually trained to do work or perform tasks for the benefit of an individual with a disability, including a physical, sensory, psychiatric, intellectual, or other mental disability." As such, students can establish their eligibility for a companion animal on campus only by having a registered service animal. The FHA's definition of "assistance animal" encompasses service animals and ESAs but does not require animals to be trained for a specific task. As such, students can submit a written physician's statement to their institution's disability center that the presence of a companion animal would benefit their mental health. Both policies recognize service animals and ESAs as disability aids, so they are both allowed in university housing that otherwise upholds a "no pets" policy. Neither policy requires accommodations be made for "pets," which are companion animals who live with a person for companionship but who are not defined as either service animals or ESAs because their owners do not have diagnosed disabilities.

There has been a fair amount of debate and confusion in the process of establishing animal-related accommodation policies at universities. As a result, even when universities comply with the ADA and FHA, the processes for approving companion animals vary significantly. Despite these variations, there has been a documented increase in ESA and service animal requests, from only 2 or 3 requests for ESAs per year in 2011 to between 60 and 75 requests per year by 2019 at Washington State University (Bauer-Wolf 2019).

The legal statutes guiding requests for companion animals exclude otherwise healthy students wishing to live with their pets—animals who could potentially act as buffers against negative mental health outcomes. Companion animal owners are "less likely to experience loneliness and depression," are more likely to feel a sense of purpose, "are less stressed by major adverse life events," and may also experience a boost in social skills because "pets are a good catalyst for meeting people" and can improve people's social interactions (Smith 2012, p. 440). Additionally, new findings suggest that enjoying the company of cats and dogs but being unable to live with one may, in fact, lead to "particularly strong depression symptoms" (Puskey and Coy 2020). Within the context of the COVID-19 pandemic, which forced many college students into online environments and greatly reduced their ability to interact with other people in person, the mental health implications of these restrictive policies became even more significant.

Conclusion

University-based AAIs are surging in use and popularity, with more than 1,000 universities worldwide providing on-campus AAIs and some universities beginning to entertain the idea of allowing companion animals on campus. Although efficacy trials on university-based AAIs are promising, characteristics of AAIs examined varied considerably by population served, type of activity, frequency and dosage of interaction offered, outcomes examined, type of animals and species incorporated, and social context in which the activity is embedded. To gain knowledge on how to best serve at-risk students, we need to conduct large randomized controlled trials using multimethod assessment approaches across multiple developmental and clinical domains, while focusing on the role of risk status in moderating treatment effects.

Key Clinical Points

- Data indicate that university students are experiencing unprecedented levels of stress, stress-related mental health symptoms, and clinical disorders.

- In response to students' overwhelming demand for psychological services and universities' limited capacity to provide services to address them, animal-assisted interventions (AAIs) can play an important *complementary* role in providing much-needed stress relief.

- AAIs are especially suitable for implementation on university campuses if they are evidence-based and tailored to the needs of the intended population.

- Universities must align their aims with selection approaches (e.g., universal, selected, or indicated), the availability and capacity of registered animal/handler teams, and the nature of risk in the student population on campus.

- If we do not examine whether treatment effects are moderated by students' risk status, we may inadvertently overlook the possibility that effective stress relief in a universal intervention is obtained only by low-risk students.

- Students with significant risk factors or existing mental health problems are better served by selected and indicated approaches that provide regular opportunities for more intense or prolonged hands-on interactions.

- At-risk students' behavioral outcomes appear to improve in response to hands-on interaction combined with didactic content presentations and activities focused on academic stress management. Cognitive outcomes such as executive functioning appear to be enhanced in at-risk populations by providing hands-on interaction exclusively.

- Although the most suitable assessment approach is likely informed by the nature of the intervention, the intended population, resources available, and outcomes targeted, each approach has utility for implementation and evaluation aims.

References

American College Health Association: American College Health Association–National College Health Assessment II: Undergraduate Student Reference Group: Executive Summary, Spring 2019. American College Health Association, 2019. Available at: https://www.acha.org/documents/ncha/NCHA-II_SPRING_2019_UNDERGRADUATE_REFERENCE%20_GROUP_EXECUTIVE_SUMMARY.pdf. Accessed August 22, 2021.

American College Health Association: American College Health Association–National College Health Assessment III: Undergraduate Student Reference Group: Executive Summary, Fall 2019. American College Health Association, 2020. Available at: https://www.acha.org/documents/ncha/NCHA-III_Fall_2019_Undergraduate_Reference_Group_Executive_Summary_updated.pdf. Accessed August 22, 2021.

American College Health Association: American College Health Association–National College Health Assessment III: Undergraduate Student Reference Group: Executive Summary, Spring 2021. American College Health Association, 2021. Available at: https://www.acha.org/documents/ncha/NCHA-III_spring-2021_undergraduate_reference_group_executive_summary_updated.pdf. Accessed September 17, 2021.

Americans With Disabilities Act, 42 U.S.C. § 12101, 1990. Available at: https://www.ada.gov/pubs/adastatute08.htm. Accessed April 25, 2021.

Bauer-Wolf J: Dog days in dorms. Inside Higher Ed, May 21, 2019. Available at: https://www.insidehighered.com/news/2019/05/21/colleges-see-rise-popularity-emotional-support-animals. Accessed July 23, 2021.

Beck AT, Steer RA: Beck Anxiety Inventory Manual, 2nd Edition. San Antonio, TX, Psychological Corporation, 1993

Beck AT, Steer RA, Brown GK: Manual for the Beck Depression Inventory, 2nd Edition. San Antonio, TX, Psychological Corporation, 1996

Binfet J-T, Passmore HA, Cebry A, et al: Reducing university students' stress through a drop-in canine-therapy program. J Ment Health 27:197–204, 2018 29265945

Carr AM, Pendry P: Understanding links between college students' childhood pet ownership, attachment, and separation anxiety during the transition to college. Anthrozoos 35(1):125–142, 2022

Center for Collegiate Mental Health: Center for Collegiate Mental Health (CCMH) 2015 Annual Report (STA 15–108). State College, PA, Penn State University, 2016. Available at: https://sites.psu.edu/ccmh/files/2017/10/2015_CCMH_Report_1-18-2015-yq3vik.pdf. Accessed March 13, 2022.

Cohen S: Perceived Stress Scale. Mind Garden, 1994. Available at: http://www.mindgarden.com/documents/PerceivedStressScale.pdf. Accessed July 19, 2021.

Craske M, Wittchen U, Bogels S, et al: DSM-5 Severity Measure for Separation Anxiety Disorder—Adult. Arlington, VA, American Psychiatric Association, 2013. Available at: https://www.psychiatry.org/File%20Library/Psychiatrists/Practice/DSM/APA_DSM5_Severity-Measure-For-Separation-Anxiety-Disorder-Adult.pdf. Accessed July 19, 2021.

Eisenberg D, Lipson SK: The Healthy Minds Study: 2018–2019 Data Report. Healthy Minds Network, 2019. Available at: https://healthymindsnetwork.org/wp-content/uploads/2019/09/HMS_national-2018-19.pdf. Accessed April 15, 2021.

Fair Housing Act, 42 U.S.C. § 3601, 1988. Available at: https://www.justice.gov/crt/fair-housing-act-2. Accessed April 25, 2021.

Greer TM, Cavalhieri KE: The role of coping strategies in understanding the effects of institutional racism on mental health outcomes for African American men. J Black Psychol 45(5):405–433, 2019

Haggerty JM, Mueller MK: Animal-assisted stress reduction programs in higher education. Innov High Educ 42(5–6):379–389, 2017

Healthy Minds Network, American College Health Association: The impact of COVID-19 on college student well-being. 2020. Available at: https://www.acha.org/documents/ncha/Healthy_Minds_NCHA_COVID_Survey_Report_FINAL.pdf. Accessed September 17, 2021.

Henriques G: The college student mental health crisis (update). Psychology Today, November 2018. Available at: https://www.psychologytoday.com/us/blog/theory-knowledge/201811/the-college-student-mental-health-crisis-update. Accessed April 5, 2021.

International Association of Human-Animal Interaction Organizations: The IAHAIO Definitions for Animal Assisted Intervention and Guidelines for Wellness of Animals Involved in AAI. Seattle, WA, IAHAIO, 2018. Available at: https://iahaio.org/best-practice/white-paper-on-animal-assisted-interventions. Accessed November 20, 2020.

Jarrett MA: Attention-deficit/hyperactivity disorder (ADHD) symptoms, anxiety symptoms, and executive functioning in emerging adults. Psychol Assess 28(2):245–250, 2016 26121381

Jau J, Hodgson D: How interaction with animals can benefit mental health: a phenomenological study. Soc Work Ment Health 16(1):20–33, 2018

Lipson SK, Lattie EG, Eisenberg D: Increased rates of mental health service utilization by U.S. college students: 10-year population-level trends (2007–2017). Psychiatr Serv 70(1):60–63, 2019 30394183

Meyer TJ, Miller ML, Metzger RL, Borkovec TD: Development and validation of the Penn State Worry Questionnaire. Behav Res Ther 28(6):487–495, 1990 2076086

National Academies of Sciences, Engineering, and Medicine: Fostering Healthy Mental, Emotional, and Behavioral Development in Children and Youth: A National Agenda. Washington, DC, National Academies Press, 2019

Pendry P, Vandagriff JL: Animal visitation program (AVP) reduces cortisol levels of university students: a randomized controlled trial. AERA Open 5(2):1–12, 2019

Pendry P, Vandagriff JL, Carr AM: Clinical depression moderates effects of animal-assisted stress prevention program on college students' emotion. J Public Ment Health 18(2):94–101, 2019

Pendry P, Carr AM, Gee NR, Vandagriff JL: Randomized trial examining effects of animal assisted intervention and stress related symptoms on college students' learning and study skills. Int J Environ Res Public Health 17(6):1909, 2020 32183453

Pendry P, Carr AM, Vandagriff JL, Gee NR: Incorporating human–animal interaction into academic stress management programs: effects on typical and at-risk college students' executive function. AERA Open 7(1):1–18, 2021

Puskey JL, Coy AE: Exploring the effects of pet preference, presence, and personality on depression symptoms. Anthrozoos 33(5):643–657, 2020

Reinecke MA: Depression: A Practitioner's Guide to Comparative Treatments (Comparative Treatment Series). Edited by Reinecke M, Davison M. New York, Springer, 2006

Sahu K, Gupta D: Life skills and mental health. Indian J Health Wellbeing 4(1):76–79, 2013

Smith B: The "pet effect"—health related aspects of companion animal ownership. Aust Fam Physician 41(6):439–442, 2012 22675689

Snyder HR: Major depressive disorder is associated with broad impairments on neuropsychological measures of executive function: a meta-analysis and review. Psychol Bull 139(1):81–132, 2013 22642228

Snyder HR, Kaiser RH, Whisman MA, et al: Opposite effects of anxiety and depressive symptoms on executive function: the case of selecting among competing options. Cogn Emotion 28(5):893–902, 2014 24295077

Son C, Hegde S, Smith A, et al: Effects of COVID-19 on college students' mental health in the United States: interview survey study. J Med Internet Res 22(9):e21279, 2020 32805704

15

Dog Visitation Programs in Hospitals

Nancy R. Gee, Ph.D.
Lisa D. Townsend, Ph.D., LCSW
Tushar P. Thakre, M.D., Ph.D.

THE PROCESS OF THE domestication of the modern dog, through active selection, has taken place over tens of thousands of years (Thalmann et al. 2013). Through this process, dogs have become adept at socializing with humans. They are sensitive to our emotional states (Albuquerque et al. 2016) and social gestures (Hare et al. 2002), able to communicate using complex cues, and able to form complex attachment relationships with humans (Miklósi et al. 2003). We now know that dogs emerged from wolves by adapting to human social demands over a period of at least 35,000 years, and there is probably no other species on the planet as well matched to human social needs as dogs (Thalmann et al. 2013). Through this lengthy selection process, many different breeds of dogs are now recognized by the American Kennel Club (see www.akc.org/dog-breeds), coming in all shapes and sizes, colors, and temperaments. Some were bred for specific behaviors or tasks like hunting or herding, whereas others were bred for the way they look or for their size or their neotenous features (Figure 15–1). Evidence indicates that people select their dogs based not on function but rather on fashion and perceived

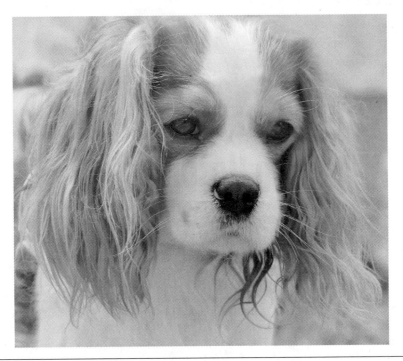

Figure 15–1.   **Examples of neotenous features in dogs.**

Features include a proportionately large forehead with lower-set, large eyes; a small nose, mouth, and chin; and a rounder, less angular face. The Cavalier King Charles spaniel embodies these features.

Source.   Image available at: https://pxhere.com/en/photo/ 539748?utm_content=shareClip&utm_medium=referral&utm_source=pxhere. The image is released free of copyrights under Creative Commons CC0.

popularity (Ghirlanda et al. 2013) or cuteness (Thorn et al. 2015). Certain physical characteristics, such as cuteness, make dogs intrinsically more appealing to humans, and humans in turn perceive cuter dogs as having more desirable personality traits (Thorn et al. 2015).

Serpell (2019) summarizes a lengthy historical perspective on animal-assisted interventions (AAIs) that includes topics such as animal souls and spiritual healing; animal powers and shamanism; animism in classical and medieval times; animals as agents of socialization, relaxation, and social support; and the roles of animals in psychotherapy. In this last-mentioned context, scientific medicine of the early decades of the twentieth century excluded animals from medical contexts. They were only mentioned in the literature in reference to zoonotic disease transmission or public health concerns. Change away from this perspective was initiated by a groundbreaking study conducted in 1980 by Friedmann and colleagues, who found that people who had been admitted to a cardiac care unit and diagnosed with myocardial infarction or angina pectoris were significantly more likely to be alive 1 year later if they owned a pet than if they did not (Friedmann et al. 1980). This finding prompted a flurry of research on, and discussion about, the importance of companion animals in human health and well-being. The preponderance of this evidence and discussion points to companion animals as a source of social support and relaxation with several short-term, relaxing effects related to animal interaction, as well as some long-term health benefits associated with pet ownership (Serpell 2019). The likely neurochemical mechanisms underlying these effects also have been identified. This body of work has given the medical community cause to reconsider the earlier exclusion of animals from hospital settings and to begin to embrace those animals as part of a vibrant and holistic approach to human health care.

There is clearly reason to suspect that including dogs in hospital settings for a variety of populations may have beneficial effects. In this chapter, we present a top-line summary of the current knowledge on dogs in hospital settings. We discuss special circumstances related to patients' service dogs, and risks associated with bringing dogs into hospital settings, and describe ways of mitigating those risks. We describe lessons learned during the coronavirus SARS-CoV-2 disease (COVID-19) pandemic and summarize the current state of science on dog visitation programs. We then present a model dog visitation program. Finally, we provide specific recommendations for practitioners about how they may take best advantage of dog visitation programs.

Potential Benefits of Dogs in Hospital Settings

Dog visitation programs in hospital settings are becoming much more popular, as evidenced by results of a survey showing that 90% of hospitals in Ontario, Canada, allow dogs to visit patients (Lefebvre et al. 2006). Many U.S. hospitals have formally integrated therapy dogs into their patient care programs (Horowitz 2010). Such programs have been associated with numerous positive outcomes for children, older adults, and people with psychiatric illnesses (Bert et al. 2016). Some of the physical and mental health benefits to patients include distraction from pain, reduced loneliness and anxiety (Nepps et al. 2014), improved ambulation (Abate et al. 2011), higher self-esteem (Chu et al. 2009), positive emotions (Caprilli and Messeri 2006), and decreased psychological distress (Gagnon et al. 2004).

Health care workers represent another important hospital population that can benefit from visits with therapy animals. Potential benefits for health care workers include reduction in biomarkers commonly associated with stress (Barker et al. 2005), decreased subjective stress, and improved social interactions with patients (Abrahamson et al. 2016). Studies have reported a reduction in salivary cortisol levels with AAIs in nurses in highly stressful work environments such as long-term care (Machová et al. 2019), as well as in emergency medicine providers (Kline et al. 2020). Similar reductions in salivary cortisol levels to those with AAI have been seen in a military population with PTSD (Rodriguez et al. 2018).

Many people assume that children in particular are likely to benefit from dog visitation programs in hospital settings. Although AAIs for hospitalized pediatric patients as a strategy for reducing physical and psychological distress have been understudied, some evidence suggests that they may be effective. Existing studies indicate that parents, nurses (Gagnon et al. 2004), and children (Caprilli and Messeri 2006) perceive canine-assisted interventions positively. Other work suggests that AAIs are associated with decreased blood pressure (Tsai et al. 2010) and self-reported pain in children who are hospitalized (Braun et al. 2009; Sobo et al. 2006).

Service Dogs in Hospitals

Service dogs pose a special set of challenges when their handler is the patient (Muramatsu et al. 2015). This situation involves balancing the rights of an individual with a disability under the Americans With Disabilities Act (ADA) and the need to provide appropriate medical care. Once the decision has been made to admit the patient to the hospital, the hospital administrators must decide whether their service dog should be admitted with them. Individuals with psychiatric service dogs may not want to be separated from their dogs, and doing so may be detrimental to the treatment process. Although no criteria have been established for determining whether an assistance dog should be admitted with the patient, Muramatsu et al. (2015) suggested substituting the term *assistance device* for *assistance animal* to help objectively determine whether the dog should be admitted with the patient. For example, if a person who uses a cane to help them walk were admitted to a psychiatric unit, is that person likely to use that device (the cane) to harm themselves or others? Similarly, suicidal patients should not be provided with a dog leash to walk their assistance dogs when they may use the leash to hang themselves. Each patient's situation is unique, and any decisions to admit a service dog with a patient to a psychiatric unit should include a risk-benefit analysis.

Next, the setting must be assessed for potential harm to others in the unit. For example, are there immunocompromised patients or other vulnerable patients in the immediate area who may be exposed to zoonotic diseases? (Please refer to the following section, "Risk Assessment and Infection Prevention.") Whether the patient is admitted with or without their dog, it should be clarified who will be responsible for the dog's care. In some cases, this will mean identifying local boarding or veterinary care facilities that may care for the dog during the patient's hospitalization. If the dog is approved to stay in the hospital with the patient, the dog should have documentation of a routine wellness examination by a veterinarian, vaccination records showing current status on all vaccinations, and a negative fecal test within the past 12 months. A protocol should be established to educate staff on hand hygiene and specific behaviors around the dog.

The patient should be made aware of their responsibility regarding property damage related to the dog and their own liability for any injury to the dog while in the hospital. The ADA clearly indicates that the handler alone is responsible for the dog. However, given that the handler is also a patient who may be unable to care for the dog at times (e.g., they may be having a sterile procedure done in a separate location in the hospital), consideration must be given to the dog's care during these times and a specific plan put into place. For example, the dog may be placed in a dog kennel/crate in the patient's room for those times when the patient must be away from the dog (e.g., in a sterile room), assuming that when the patient returns to their room, they can then care for the dog again. If the patient's ability to care for the dog is in question, an alternative person must be on hand to take care of the dog, or the dog must be cared for outside the hospital.

Risk Assessment and Infection Prevention

Hospital policies vary widely with regard to implementation of health requirements for therapy animals (Linder et al. 2017). The American Veterinary Medical Association (2022a) offers guidelines for initiating AAIs in health care facilities, including recommendations for mitigating risk of zoonotic illness transmission. In addition, the Society for Healthcare Epidemiology of America offers guidelines for infection prevention in the context of hospital-based animal-assisted activities (Murthy et al. 2015). For a detailed "how to" guide to setting up a dog visitation program in a health care setting, we suggest *Animal-Assisted Interventions in Health Care Settings: A Best Practices Manual for Establishing New Programs* by Barker et al. (2019). This manual and the procedures described therein serve as the foundation for the best practices example program we discuss in this chapter, but first, it is important to discuss potential risks and how to mitigate them.

Potential Risks and How to Ameliorate Those Risks

Controlling the transmission of disease is of paramount importance in a health care setting, and zoonotic disease transmission is a key concern when the implementation of a dog visitation program is being considered. Ameliorating the risk of zoonotic disease transmission should not be taken lightly, but it is not terribly complicated to accomplish. It is important to keep dogs out of respiratory isolation rooms where patients have or are suspected to have tuberculosis, because although dogs are resistant to human tuberculosis, they can transmit the disease to humans (Hardy 1981). The already low risk potential for the zoonotic transmission of bacterial infections such as *Escherichia coli*, salmonellae, staphylococcus, or streptococcus can be reduced or eliminated by handwashing, before and after touching the dog, by preventing dogs with open wounds from visiting the hospital, and by preventing humans with uncovered open wounds from interacting with dogs. A study examining the presence of various types of bacteria on the soles of people's shoes, pet dog paws, and assistance dog paws found that dog paws had significantly lower bacterial counts than did the soles of shoes and that there was no significant difference in bacterial counts between pet dog paws and assistance dog paws (Vos et al. 2021). The authors concluded that dog paws in general have better hygiene than shoe soles.

Hardy (1981) suggested that dog visitation should not take place when the patient is in isolation for respiratory, enteric, or other infectious diseases, or in reverse isolation; is immunocompromised or has an immunocompromised roommate; or has a severe allergy to, or phobia of, dogs. Dogs also should not visit patients who may be experiencing active symptoms of psychosis or showing signs of agitation or aggressive behavior, or who have a service dog in the room, or when someone else in the room has a service dog present. Finally, Lefebvre et al. (2006) presented data that suggest that routine screening for *Salmonella* species and *Giar-*

dia species may be warranted, but they also indicated that appropriate infection control procedures may reduce the risk of pathogen transmission.

Lessons Learned From COVID-19

Most hospital-based therapy dog programs in the United States were placed on hiatus during the months following the initial outbreak of COVID-19. On further evaluation of COVID-19 virus transmission vectors, the U.S. Centers for Disease Control and Prevention (CDC) concluded that the risk of viral transmission from animals to humans is low and that no evidence indicates that animal skin or fur is a vector for infection (Centers for Disease Control and Prevention 2022; see also American Veterinary Medical Association 2022c). Worldwide, only 81 dogs and 115 cats have been documented to be infected with COVID-19 (American Veterinary Medical Association 2022b). Those infections have occurred under conditions of close contact between the animals and the humans who tested positive for COVID-19. No evidence has found that canines or felines who are positive for COVID-19 serve as transmission vectors to humans (American Veterinary Medical Association 2022b; Centers for Disease Control and Prevention 2021a). Therefore, routine testing of animals for the virus is not recommended (American Veterinary Medical Association 2011).

Guidelines for therapy animal visits established by the CDC include handwashing by handlers before and after visits, avoiding visiting known COVID-positive patients, social distancing between humans not involved in the interaction, not allowing animals to lick people, and using masks and face shields on humans. The guidelines note that masks and disinfecting agents, such as hand sanitizer, should not be used on animals (Centers for Disease Control and Prevention 2021b).

In summary, no evidence indicates that dogs can transmit the COVID-19 virus to humans. Although many therapy dog visitation programs were halted during the first year of the COVID-19 pandemic, it appears that dogs can safely visit patients. The primary concern for preventing transmission of COVID-19 is that the human handlers wear appropriate personal protective equipment and follow sanitation protocols before and after interacting with patients. Aside from COVID-19, however, other zoonoses well known to veterinary and medical professionals can be transmitted from therapy dogs to humans. These transmissions can be prevented through appropriate vaccination schedules and grooming as well as by using physical barriers on surfaces that come into contact with animal paws (American Veterinary Medical Association 2011).

With proper attention to infection prevention protocols, therapy animals can safely visit hospitalized patients.

Scientific Evidence Base

Other chapters in this book have summarized the existing evidence on how companion animals may be beneficial in the treatment process for disorders or illnesses that may require hospitalization, such as in the context of depression (Chapter 8), crisis intervention (Chapter 4), PTSD (Chapter 10), autism spectrum disorder (Chapter 7), serious mental illness (Chapter 11), and palliative care (Chapter 12). Rather than summarize that evidence here, we focus on and highlight examples and evidence regarding the efficacy of dog visitation programs that are unique to hospital settings.

Examples of Dog Visitation in Hospital Settings

Waiting Rooms

Therapy dogs can provide a source of comfort and distraction for patients awaiting outpatient procedures and their families, or for families of those patients undergoing more extensive surgical procedures. Certain outpatient procedures, such as infusions, dialysis, and diagnostic procedures, can be lengthy and associated with boredom or anxiety. Therapy dogs can mitigate some of the stress that accompanies long periods of waiting for patients and loved ones (Miller and Ingram 2000).

Emergency Departments

Patients who present to the emergency department are often experiencing significant pain and anxiety, and these symptoms are potentially exacerbated by long wait times. Therapy dogs can provide invaluable support to patients and families who are waiting for or receiving care. One randomized controlled trial evaluated the efficacy of a therapy dog visit compared with treatment as usual for emergency department patients struggling with acute anxiety; findings indicated significant improvement in anxiety symptoms for the therapy dog visit group (Kline et al. 2019).

Inpatient Units

Therapy dogs can visit most hospital units if appropriate risk assessment and risk management are in place. In one model evidence-based program (Barker and Gee 2021), dogs can visit everywhere in the hospital except for surgical suites and locations where food is being served. Therapy dog visits are associated with pain reduction on orthopedic units (Harper et al. 2015), decreased depression symptoms on oncology units (Orlandi et al. 2007), improved mood and motivation on burn units (Pruskowski et al. 2020), and reduced anxiety among hospitalized pediatric patients (Hinic et al. 2019).

Health Care Worker Support

Therapy dog support for health care workers remains an underexplored area of AAI research. Preliminary studies of health care workers' response to the presence of therapy dogs suggested that these workers perceive significant benefit from interacting with animals in the workplace (Abrahamson et al. 2016) and showed significant reductions in stress biomarkers following brief interactions with a dog (Barker et al. 2005). These findings suggest that AAI delivered in an ultrabrief format may alleviate stress in health care workers (Figure 15–2). Animal-assisted programs also have been suggested as a potential way to reduce burnout among health care workers and improve their job perception and mental health (Etingen et al. 2020; Jensen et al. 2021).

Evaluation of the Evidence Base

A common refrain in the field of human-animal interaction is that more high-quality research is needed to fully understand when, where, and how dog interaction may be beneficial. Although we know that even brief therapy dog visits can lead to positive health results via mechanisms including reductions in stress hormones, increases in endorphin and oxytocin levels, reduction in blood pressure, and activation of mirror neurons (Marcus 2013), we do not fully understand what characteristics of the interaction are important to accruing any potential benefits. For example, is it necessary to touch the dog to benefit, or can people watch the dog? Is it more likely to be beneficial for people who own, or have owned, pets or dogs? We have some preliminary answers to these questions, but the studies tend to use different methodologies and the results are mixed, so it is challenging to draw meaningful conclusions without more high-quality research. Furthermore, research that includes longitudinal follow-up is needed to assess whether effects of AAI are durable once an individual returns home (Chur-Hansen et al. 2014).

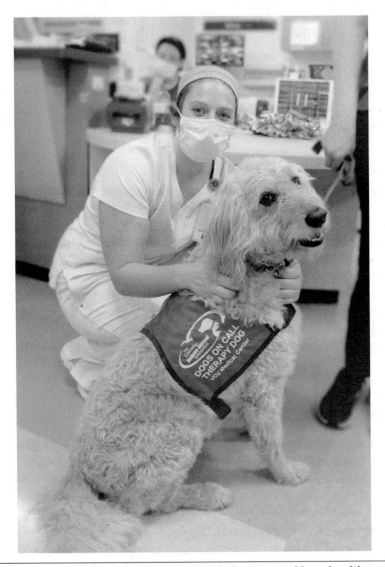

Figure 15–2.   Dogs on Call therapy dog being greeted by a health care worker at Virginia Commonwealth University Medical Center.

Source.   Photograph provided courtesy of the Center for Human-Animal Interaction, School of Medicine, Virginia Commonwealth University.

Best Practices Example Program

Dogs on Call

The Dogs on Call (DOC) program in the Center for Human-Animal Interaction (CHAI) at Virginia Commonwealth University was established in 2001. It is the only center of its kind housed in a school of medicine (other such centers tend to be housed in veterinary schools), and thus it is intimately incorporated into a major metropolitan health system (Center for Human-Animal Interaction 2021). CHAI's mission is improving health and well-being through human-animal interaction. Prior to the pandemic, there were nearly 100 DOC teams, consisting of a human volunteer and a therapy dog registered with either Pet Partners or Alliance of Therapy Dogs. Teams visit throughout the hospital, providing comfort to pediatric and adult patients, health care workers and staff, and visitors. In addition, DOC teams provide stress relief at organized wellness events for students, faculty, and staff, such as visiting the student center during final examinations week or providing relief for health care workers after a difficult loss. More information about CHAI and its therapy dog teams is available on the center's website (https://chai.vcu.edu).

Animal Welfare

A key component of the DOC program involves ensuring the well-being of all therapy dogs who volunteer at the hospital. All DOC therapy dogs receive regular veterinary and behavioral evaluations to assess their physical health and suitability for volunteering in a busy hospital environment. Veterinary records are updated yearly, including required vaccinations, negative fecal examinations, and a successful wellness examination signed by the veterinarians. CHAI staff members with animal behavior experience shadow teams on hospital visits yearly to assess changes in the dogs' responses to potential stressors they may encounter while visiting. Dogs are permitted to visit the hospital for a maximum of 2 hours each day; this requirement helps to limit any physical and mental stress that the therapy dogs may experience during their time in the hospital.

Dog visitation in a hospital may be accompanied by several sights, sounds, and smells that are harsh and potentially repulsive or scary to the dog, so it is important to limit their exposure by strictly adhering to the 2-hour time limit. Dogs also need time to habituate to common hospital sights, sounds, and smells. To accomplish this, CHAI provides opportunities for DOC handlers to practice visitation with their dogs in a part of the hospital that primarily houses office staff. Although this area is not identical to the parts of the hospital that perform patient care, it has similar flooring, elevators, and lighting, and many of the same sounds. Handlers may, for example, bring their dogs and some treats and practice rewarding the dogs for riding in the elevators, because elevators can initially be frightening to inexperienced dogs. The treats can make the elevator ride a positive experience for the dogs, and the experience provides an example of how CHAI helps DOC handlers prepare their dogs for successful and low-stress hospital visitation.

Handlers

Most DOC team handlers are registered volunteers at Virginia Commonwealth University (VCU) Health, with a smaller percentage being employee handlers. All handlers undergo a rigorous background check, fingerprinting, Health Insurance Portability and Accountability Act training, and orientation to hospital safety and privacy practices before being evaluated for DOC. CHAI provides ongoing animal welfare education to handlers, and some teams deliver AAIs for research studies. In most dog visitation programs, volunteer handlers have limited previous exposure to the stress and emotional upset they may experience while visiting patients in the hospital. Handlers need support to process the extreme emotional situations they may witness, such as providing comfort to a family while they cope with the death of a loved one or visiting with a child receiving chemotherapy. CHAI provides ongoing education to handlers to help them develop strategies for managing conflicting demands on their time and emotional resources. For example, DOC teams are limited to 2 hours in the hospital on a given day, but the handler may hesitate to the leave the bedside of a sick patient because the patient or a family member has asked them to stay. CHAI provides strategies for exiting a situation as gracefully as possible, while also arranging for another DOC team to come visit the patient. Furthermore, DOC handlers must divide their attention between the needs of their dog and the demands of the environment. They sometimes need to navigate loud and crowded hallways, or respond to a health care worker's urgent request, but in so doing, they must always place the needs of their dog first. DOC handlers are trained to recognize signs of stress in their dog and to act quickly to remove the dog from the source of stress. Sometimes this means taking the dog outside for a quick break or cutting their time in the hospital short and leaving for the day. It is important to keep the dogs calm and happy about visiting so that they will want to keep coming back. A dog who does not enjoy the work will not be as effective and may ultimately refuse to continue to be a therapy dog.

Program Evaluation and Popularity

In the full year immediately prior to the pandemic, DOC teams engaged in more than 91,000 meaningful (more than 3-minute-long) human-animal interactions. In a quality assurance patient satisfaction survey of 407 patients, 99% of them reported that the DOC visits were helpful. Patients provided reasons such as improved mood and reduced loneliness, depression, and anxiety, and some patients even reported reduced pain (Figure 15–3). Nursing staff collect and post DOC team trading cards with pictures of the dogs at their stations. They also frequently request DOC wellness visits or visits from DOC teams when the staff are particularly vulnerable to compassion fatigue or burnout. Anecdotally, the staff report that DOC visits make their day and help them to keep doing what they do. The pandemic has driven these types of anecdotal reports to an all-time high. In fact, the DOC teams are so popular that when they returned to visitation following the introduction of the COVID-19 vaccines, the teams needed escorts to help all of their adoring fans adhere to social distancing requirements in the hospital.

Case Example: Future Veterinarian Survives Cancer With the Help of Some Furry Friends

"Dr. Eric" was just 10 years old when he was diagnosed with acute lymphoblastic leukemia, setting him on a 3-year journey to battle the illness. An animal lover before leukemia struck, Eric was befriended by several DOC therapy dogs who supported him at the hospital during his lengthy treatment. His new friends included a Maltese named Stewie and a Yorkshire terrier called Winnie. He defeated leukemia and prepared to embark on another journey—this time to become a veterinarian to care for animals just like they cared for him.

Key Clinical Points

- Handlers and dogs must be trained to cope with the unique circumstances often found in hospital settings: sights, sounds, smells, and the emotions of patients, families, and staff.

- It is essential to establish and adhere to animal welfare guidelines in all aspects of such hospital work; this is

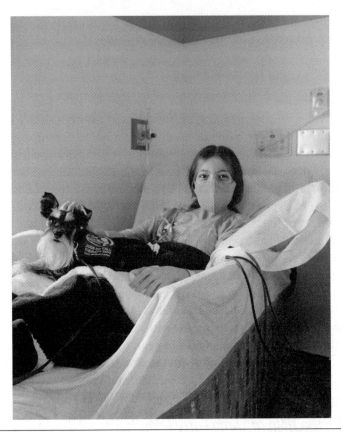

Figure 15–3.   A patient receives a visit from a Dogs on Call therapy dog.

Note how a barrier (towel) is used between the dog and the patient's bedding, the leash is always on the dog and (outside the picture frame) in the handler's hand, and the dog is situated in a way that will reduce close face-to-face contact with the patient.

Source.   Photograph provided courtesy of the Center for Human-Animal Interaction, School of Medicine, Virginia Commonwealth University.

not only humane but also likely to result in a more effective therapy dog.

- Those responsible for therapy dog programs in hospitals must regularly review the human-animal interaction literature to maintain their knowledge about evidence-based animal-assisted intervention practices and distinguish valid evidence from popular opinion.
- The recent COVID-19 pandemic has highlighted the need to consult with infectious disease experts when

faced with novel illnesses to determine the effect on any therapy animal visitation program.

References

Abate SV, Zucconi M, Boxer BA: Impact of canine-assisted ambulation on hospitalized chronic heart failure patients' ambulation outcomes and satisfaction: a pilot study. J Cardiovasc Nurs 26(3):224–230, 2011 21263346

Abrahamson K, Cai Y, Richards E, et al: Perceptions of a hospital-based animal assisted intervention program: an exploratory study. Complement Ther Clin Pract 25:150–154, 2016 27863605

Albuquerque N, Guo K, Wilkinson A, et al: Dogs recognize dog and human emotions. Biol Lett 12(1):20150883, 2016 26763220

American Veterinary Medical Association: Guidelines for Animal-Assisted Activity, Animal-Assisted Therapy and Resident Animal Programs. Schaumberg, IL, American Veterinary Medical Association, 2011. Available at: https://ebusiness.avma.org/files/productdownloads/guidelines_AAA.pdf. Accessed November 2, 2021.

American Veterinary Medical Association: Animal assisted interventions: guidelines. Schaumberg, IL, American Veterinary Medical Association, 2022a. Available at: https://www.avma.org/resources-tools/avma-policies/animal-assisted-interventions-guidelines. Accessed January 12, 2022.

American Veterinary Medical Association: COVID-19. Schaumberg, IL, American Veterinary Medical Association, 2022b. Available at: https://www.avma.org/resources-tools/animal-health-and-welfare/covid-19. Accessed January 12, 2022.

American Veterinary Medical Association: SARS-CoV-2 in animals. Schaumberg, IL, American Veterinary Medical Association, 2022c. Available at: https://www.avma.org/resources-tools/animal-health-and-welfare/covid-19/sars-cov-2-animals-including-pets. Accessed January 12, 2022.

Barker SB, Gee NR: Canine-assisted interventions in hospitals: best practices for maximizing human and canine safety. Front Vet Sci 8:615730, 2021 33869316

Barker SB, Knisely JS, McCain NL, Best AM: Measuring stress and immune response in healthcare professionals following interaction with a therapy dog: a pilot study. Psychol Rep 96(3 Pt 1):713–729, 2005 16050629

Barker SB, Vokes RA, Barker RT: Animal-Assisted Interventions in Health Care Settings: A Best Practices Manual for Establishing New Programs. West Lafayette, IN, Purdue University Press, 2019

Bert F, Gualano MR, Camussi E, et al: Animal assisted intervention: a systematic review of benefits and risks. Eur J Integr Med 8(5):695–706, 2016 32362955

Braun C, Stangler T, Narveson J, Pettingell S: Animal-assisted therapy as a pain relief intervention for children. Complement Ther Clin Pract 15(2):105–109, 2009 19341990

Caprilli S, Messeri A: Animal-assisted activity at A. Meyer Children's Hospital: a pilot study. Evid Based Complement Alternat Med 3(3):379–383, 2006 16951723

Center for Human-Animal Interaction: Our mission. Richmond, Virginia Commonwealth University, 2021. Available at: https://chai.vcu.edu. Accessed November 10, 2021.

Centers for Disease Control and Prevention: Guidance for handlers of service and therapy animals. Atlanta, GA, Centers for Disease Control and Prevention, 2021a. Available at: https://www.cdc.gov/healthypets/covid-19/service-therapy-animals.html. Accessed November 2, 2021.

Centers for Disease Control and Prevention: Guidance for handlers of service and therapy animals: ways to protect therapy animals. Atlanta, GA, Centers for Disease Control and Prevention, 2021b. Available at: https://www.cdc.gov/healthypets/covid-19/service-therapy-animals.html#definitions. Accessed November 2, 2021.

Centers for Disease Control and Prevention: Frequently asked questions: pets and animals. Atlanta, GA, Centers for Disease Control and Prevention, 2022. Available at: https://www.cdc.gov/coronavirus/2019-ncov/faq.html#Pets-and-Animals. Accessed March 16, 2022.

Chu CI, Liu CY, Sun CT, Lin J: The effect of animal-assisted activity on inpatients with schizophrenia. J Psychosoc Nurs Ment Health Serv 47(12):42–48, 2009 20000282

Chur-Hansen A, McArthur M, Winefield H, et al: Animal-assisted interventions in children's hospitals: a critical review of the literature. Anthrozoos 27(1):5–18, 2014

Etingen B, Martinez RN, Smith BM, et al: Developing an animal-assisted support program for healthcare employees. BMC Health Serv Res 20(1):714, 2020 32746817

Friedmann E, Katcher AH, Lynch JJ, Thomas SA: Animal companions and one-year survival of patients after discharge from a coronary care unit. Public Health Rep 95(4):307–312, 1980 6999524

Gagnon J, Bouchard F, Landry M, et al: Implementing a hospital-based animal therapy program for children with cancer: a descriptive study. Can Oncol Nurs J 14(4):217–222, 2004 15635895

Ghirlanda S, Acerbi A, Herzog H, Serpell JA: Fashion vs. function in cultural evolution: the case of dog breed popularity. PLoS One 8(9):e74770, 2013 24040341

Hardy G: The seeing-eye dog: an infection risk in hospital? Can Med Assoc J 124(6):698–700, 1981 7171013

Hare B, Brown M, Williamson C, Tomasello M: The domestication of social cognition in dogs. Science 298(5598):1634–1636, 2002 12446914

Harper CM, Dong Y, Thornhill TS, et al: Can therapy dogs improve pain and satisfaction after total joint arthroplasty? A randomized controlled trial. Clin Orthop Relat Res 473(1):372–379, 2015 25201095

Hinic K, Kowalski MO, Holtzman K, Mobus K: The effect of a pet therapy and comparison intervention on anxiety in hospitalized children. J Pediatr Nurs 46:55–61, 2019 30852256

Horowitz S: Animal-assisted therapy for inpatients: tapping the unique healing power of the human-animal bond. Altern Complement Ther 16(6):339–343, 2010

Jensen CL, Bibbo J, Rodriguez KE, O'Haire ME: The effects of facility dogs on burnout, job-related well-being, and mental health in paediatric hospital professionals. J Clin Nurs 30(9–10):1429–1441, 2021 33555610

Kline JA, Fisher MA, Pettit KL, et al: Controlled clinical trial of canine therapy versus usual care to reduce patient anxiety in the emergency department. PLoS One 14(1):e0209232, 2019 30625184

Kline JA, VanRyzin K, Davis JC, et al: Randomized trial of therapy dogs versus deliberative coloring (art therapy) to reduce stress in emergency medicine providers. Acad Emerg Med 27(4):266–275, 2020 32266765

Lefebvre SL, Waltner-Toews D, Peregrine AS, et al: Prevalence of zoonotic agents in dogs visiting hospitalized people in Ontario: implications for infection control. J Hosp Infect 62(4):458–466, 2006 16466831

Linder DE, Siebens HC, Mueller MK, et al: Animal-assisted interventions: a national survey of health and safety policies in hospitals, eldercare facilities, and therapy animal organizations. Am J Infect Control 45(8):883–887, 2017 28673680

Machová K, Součková M, Procházková R, et al: Canine-assisted therapy improves well-being in nurses. Int J Environ Res Public Health 16(19):3670, 2019 31574899

Marcus DA: The science behind animal-assisted therapy. Curr Pain Headache Rep 17(4):322, 2013

Miklósi A, Kubinyi E, Topál J, et al: A simple reason for a big difference: wolves do not look back at humans, but dogs do. Curr Biol 13(9):763–766, 2003 12725735

Miller J, Ingram L: Perioperative nursing and animal-assisted therapy. AORN J 72(3):477–483, 2000 11004963

Muramatsu RS, Thomas KJ, Leong SL, Ragukonis F: Service dogs, psychiatric hospitalization, and the ADA. Psychiatr Serv 66(1):87–89, 2015

Murthy R, Bearman G, Brown S, et al: Animals in healthcare facilities: recommendations to minimize potential risks. Infect Control Hosp Epidemiol 36(5):495–516, 2015 25998315

Nepps P, Stewart CN, Bruckno SR: Animal-assisted activity: effects of a complementary intervention program on psychological and physiological variables. J Evid Based Complementary Altern Med 19(3):211–215, 2014 24789913

Orlandi M, Trangeled K, Mambrini A, et al: Pet therapy effects on oncological day hospital patients undergoing chemotherapy treatment. Anticancer Res 27(6C):4301–4303, 2007 18214035

Pruskowski KA, Gurney JM, Cancio LC: Impact of the implementation of a therapy dog program on burn center patients and staff. Burns 46(2):293–297, 2020 31852614

Rodriguez KE, Bryce CI, Granger DA, O'Haire ME: The effect of a service dog on salivary cortisol awakening response in a military population with posttraumatic stress disorder (PTSD). Psychoneuroendocrinology 98:202–210, 2018 29907299

Serpell J: Animal-assisted intervention in historical perspective, in Handbook on Animal-Assisted Therapy: Foundations and Guidelines for Animal-Assisted Interventions, 5th Edition. Edited by Fine AH. Cambridge, MA, Academic Press, 2019, pp 13–22

Sobo EJ, Eng B, Kassity-Krich N: Canine visitation (pet) therapy: pilot data on decreases in child pain perception. J Holist Nurs 24(1):51–57, 2006 16449747

Thalmann O, Shapiro B, Cui P, et al: Complete mitochondrial genomes of ancient canids suggest a European origin of domestic dogs. Science 342(6160):871–874, 2013 24233726

Thorn P, Howell TJ, Brown C, Bennett PC: The canine cuteness effect: owner-perceived cuteness as a predictor of human–dog relationship quality. Anthrozoos 8(4):569–585, 2015

Tsai CC, Friedmann E, Thomas SA: The effect of animal-assisted therapy on stress responses in hospitalized children. Anthrozoos 23(3):245–258, 2010

Vos SJ, Wijnker JJ, Overgaauw PA: A pilot study on the contamination of assistance dogs' paws and their users' shoe soles in relation to admittance to hospitals and (in) visible disability. Int J Environ Res Public Health 18(2):513, 2021

16

Animal-Assisted Therapy in Psychotherapy

Cynthia K. Chandler, Ed.D.

Animal-Assisted Therapy (AAT) is a method whereby the incorporation of human-animal interaction (HAI) advances the recovery of a human client. The therapeutic method of AAT is HAI. The primary therapeutic agent of AAT is a human therapist who facilitates interactions between a human client and a therapy animal who works like a secondary therapeutic agent. The value of incorporating an additional therapeutic agent, a therapy animal, and an additional therapeutic method, HAI, adds to the potential progress that can be made in psychotherapy.

Quality of Existing Evidence

Relatively little rigorous study of animal-assisted psychotherapy has been done, yet studies have shown this type of approach to be effective. For instance, Dietz et al. (2012) showed how combining therapeutic storytelling with AAT led to improvement in symptoms of sexually abused children. A total of 153 children ages 7–17 years who were in group therapy at a child advocacy center participated in their study. The researchers evaluated and compared the efficacy of three different treatments: dogs present with stories ($n=61$), dogs present with no stories ($n=60$), and stories without dogs present ($n=32$). The narrative stories were about the therapy dogs' experiences and were written specifically to coincide with the therapy topics in each session. Results indicated that children in the psychotherapy groups that included therapy dogs showed significant decreases in trauma symptoms including anxiety, depression, anger, PTSD, dissociation, and sexual concerns. All three groups showed significant improvement in trauma symptoms, but the dogs present with stories group showed the most change, the stories without dogs present group showed the second most improvement, and the group with dogs present but without stories showed the least improvement. The results of this study suggested that including therapy dogs with a psychotherapeutic approach (in this case, storytelling) was the most effective.

Another example of clinical efficacy of animal-assisted psychotherapy is a study by Trotter et al. (2008), performed with 164 elementary- and middle-school children identified as at risk for academic and social failure. This study showed the efficacy of equine-assisted counseling by comparing it with an established, award-winning classroom-based group counseling curriculum that did not involve animals. Equine-assisted counseling consisted of 12 weekly small group counseling sessions (eight members each). Each 3-hour session involved participants interacting with horses in various structured and semistructured exercises designed to facilitate trust-building, enhance social and relational skills, and increase emotion recognition and regulation. A comparison of within-group pre- and posttreatment scores determined that the equine-assisted counseling group ($n=126$, target group) had significant improvement in 17 behavior areas, including child self-reports of emotional symptoms, clinical maladjustment, atypical behaviors, sense of inadequacy, and relationships with parents and parent reports of the child's behavioral symptoms, internalizing problems, externalizing problems, adaptive skills, hyperactivity, aggression, conduct problems, anxiety, depression, somatization, adaptability, and social skills. The classroom-based counseling group ($n=38$, comparison group) showed significant improvement in only five areas, and four of these five were different areas: child self-reports of emotional symptoms, personal adjustment, social stress, and self-esteem and parent reports of the child's depression. Between-group results indicated that equine-assisted counseling was superior to classroom-based counseling, with significantly greater improvement in seven areas when the two treatments were compared directly. Furthermore, repeated-measures analysis of equine-assisted counseling participants' social behavior ratings on a psychosocial measure completed after each session showed significant improvement, with increases in positive behaviors and decreases in negative behaviors (Trotter et al. 2008).

Bachi et al. (2012) reported positive effects of equine-facilitated individual psychotherapy with at-risk adolescents at a residential treatment facility. Fourteen resident adolescents made up the treatment group and were compared with a matched group of 15 residents who did not receive the equine-facilitated psychotherapy (control). The treatment consisted of a weekly 50-minute equine-facilitated individual psychotherapy session offered over a period of 7 months. Interventions included touching and grooming the horse to make a social connection and riding the horse for a physical dimension to facilitate the establishment of a healthy physical self-image and the healing of the damaged emotional and sensory motor elements. The study found a trend of positive change in all four research parameters within the treatment group: self-image, self-control, trust, and general life satisfaction (Bachi et al. 2012).

Prothmann et al. (2006) used a pretest-posttest design to investigate possible influences of AAT incorporating the presence of a therapy dog on the state of mind of children and adolescents who have undergone inpatient psychiatric treatment. State of mind was defined as vitality, intraemotional balance, social extroversion, and alertness. A total of 100 children and adolescents, ages 11–20 years, who were undergoing inpatient child and adolescent psychiatric treatment participated in this study. Sixty-one children and adolescents (Group 1 treatment group) participated in AAT during their inpatient stay. Thirty-nine children were put into a comparison group (Group 2) and did not receive AAT. The "dog therapy" was conducted as a nondirected, free-play therapy. Each child participated in five weekly sessions during which a certified therapy dog was available for 30 minutes (five sessions over 5 weeks). There were no direct instructions regulating the course of the therapy; the participants were free to choose the kind of interaction they had with the dog (e.g., playing, stroking, cuddling, feeding). The same toys were available to each person, and everybody was motivated to interact with the dog. Nobody ignored the animal. For Group 1 patients, the pre- and posttest results showed highly significant increases in all dimensions of state of mind. These changes were not found in Group 2 patients. Researchers concluded that incorporating a dog into therapy sessions could catalyze psychotherapeutic work with children and adolescents (Prothmann et al. 2006). Given that the incorporation of therapy animals has been shown to be effective at enriching the psychotherapy process, it is relevant to explore why and how this may occur.

Relational Value of Animals Participating in Psychotherapy

Humans and other mammals have similar biological systems for within-species and across-species social engagement: the social response system and the stress response system (Daley Olmert 2009; Odendaal 2000; Odendaal and Meintjes 2003; Panksepp 2004, 2005). It is important to understand how these two separate yet interconnected and interactive systems are involved in animal-assisted psychotherapy. The thrive system, which involves reward and gratification, is the social response system. Mammals are wired to attend to themselves and others through social interaction. They commonly seek out social interaction for comfort and nurturance and as a way of reducing stress in themselves or another. The survive system, often referred to as the fight-flight-freeze response, is the stress response system. When humans and other mammals perceive a reason to be distressed, stress-related hormones such as aldosterone, cortisol, and adrenaline are then released into the body, resulting in fight, flight, or freeze responses (Panksepp 2004, 2005). These responses are maintained until the human or animal no longer perceives a reason to be distressed.

Thus, animals can experience distress from negative social interaction in much the same way as humans. Moreover, when the animal's behavior reflects this in response to a person, the animal's behavior serves as a mirror to an individual, perhaps reflecting either a client's attitude and behavior or those of a session facilitator.

An animal may serve in the role of "emotional distress detector" for human participants during HAI via behaviors initiated from activation of the stress response system (Chandler 2017). Many species of animals will demonstrate calming signals, alerting signals, or displacement signals when the animal experiences stress or perceives distress in another being (Chandler 2017; Rugaas 2005). All of these are naturally occurring animal behaviors. Examples of calming signals of dogs include looking away, yawning, rapid lip licking, rapid eye blinking, sniffing the ground, or a quick shake of the body (Chandler 2017; Rugaas 2005). Other species have similar calming signals, as well as some that are different. Horses demonstrate many of the same signals as dogs and also may engage in behaviors such as empty chewing or pawing the ground (Chandler 2017). Alerting signals of animals are behaviors or expressions, either vocal or nonvocal, that may direct attention (Chandler 2017). Alerting signals include a dog pacing back and forth between therapist and client, a dog barking quickly and briefly, a dog or a horse staring in one direction with ears up and forward, a horse whinnying or snorting, and a horse repeatedly motioning its head in a certain direction. Displacement signals of animals include moving away, moving toward, or some other major shift in body position or posture (Chandler 2017).

The social response systems of humans and other mammals are also similar. Within a few minutes of the initiation of positive social interaction with a therapy animal, levels of human hormones associated with the experience of well-being (e.g., dopamine, endorphins, and oxytocin) will rise (Odendaal 2000; Odendaal and Meintjes 2003). This is a social response reward mechanism, meaning that a social interaction feels good or is rewarding. Dopamine stimulates the pleasure centers in the brain, endorphins lift mood, and oxytocin stimulates social connection, enhances mood, and suppresses the stress response system, thereby inducing a calming effect. Furthermore, the effects of oxytocin are enhanced when positive touch occurs during social interaction (i.e., petting an animal), causing skin sensors to stimulate the release of substantial amounts of oxytocin in the brain (Handlin et al. 2011; Uvänas-Moberg et al. 2005). Animals such as dogs and horses can experience interaction and contact with humans as nurturing in much the same way (Panksepp 2004, 2005). The social response reward mechanism underlies an animal's desire to seek and provide engagement that can be very beneficial to a client. Via activation of the social response system, an animal may serve in the role of "nurturer" for human participants during HAI; likewise, a human participant is provided an opportunity to serve as "nurturer" for the animal (Chandler 2017).

Significant Human–Animal Relational Moments

HAI is affected by the perception of sensory stimuli in the environment and motivational processing via neural pathways for thrive and survive needs in the brain that contribute to behaviors. From the moment a therapy animal and human enter each other's perceptual field, they each begin to gather information through sensory perception about potential thrive rewards and whether any indicators are present that suggest a need to act for survival preservation. Perceived stimuli are also compared with previous learned experiences to assist in making determinations about the current situation. Thus, HAI is a complex neurobiological event.

HAI manifests as a series of relational moments that are occurring in both humans and animals when they are in each other's perceptual fields (Chandler 2017, 2018). Some of these relational moments can be more impactful than others. The impact will be specific to the wants, needs, and desires of both the animal and the human in the relational experience. A facilitator who is highly trained and experienced in the complexities of HAI will be able to mostly understand what humans and animals are experiencing and communicating and then more effectively facilitate a session for better outcome. With a plethora of relational moments occurring during HAI, it is most useful during an AAT session to focus on the relational moment or moments that are most pronounced and have greatest potential for therapeutic effect. These are referred to as *significant human-animal relational moments*; this construct comes from the model known as human-animal relational theory (Chandler 2018).

When HAI is incorporated into psychotherapy, additional opportunities for therapeutic gain can emerge. This is primarily due to increased psychodynamics—that is, an increase in the motivational forces, both conscious and unconscious, that may surface in an AAT session. Vital particulars of the psychodynamic process include the relational experiences of those involved, experiences facilitated by a therapist and processed with a client. In AAT, therapists perform types of individual and group processes that are similar to those that they are trained to perform in non-AAT sessions. However, when HAIs are incorporated as they are in AAT, there are more particulars made available to the therapist and client to experience, increasing and enhancing opportunities to affect human attitudes and behaviors. Numerous relational experiences are involved in AAT: the therapist's experience of the client and the client's experience of the therapist with the therapy animal observing; the client's experience of the therapy animal along with the therapy animal's experience of the client with the therapist observing; and the therapist's experience of the therapy animal along with the therapy animal's experience of the therapist with the client observing. Interactions might happen consecutively or concurrently; for example, a client and therapist both might be interacting with a therapy animal at the same time. Each of these interactions provides opportunities for meaningful experience for the parties involved. These experiences may reveal for the therapist and the client important motivational forces of the client.

A therapy animal can serve in two primary relational roles during AAT: nurturer and emotional distress detector. Domesticated animals that are mammals commonly seek out social interaction for comfort and nurturance, including being close in proximity, being touched or petted, or engaging in play. They also behave in ways that reflect stress or attempts to cope with stress. For instance, mammals are neurologically wired to detect and respond to stress by 1) signaling an alert when in need or alarm in the presence of threat, 2) moving toward another to receive comfort, 3) moving toward a stressed other so as to provide comfort or to nurture, and 4) moving away from a stressor for self-care or self-preservation. Through their senses, animals detect and then respond to what they perceive in their environment. For instance, the sophisticated olfactory system of dogs and horses (Rørvang et al. 2020; Singletary and Lazarowski 2021) allows them to detect emotions from human body excretions (Filiatre et al. 1991) and then respond in ways that may reflect the internal emotional state of a client.

An AAT facilitator must be well trained in the interpretation of animal body language and communication to recognize their meaning and significance in a session. An animal's behavior can provide information to a therapist that might not otherwise be revealed without the presence of the animal. A key in correctly interpreting an animal's communication is to place the animal's behavior in context within a session. For instance, a therapist must attempt to discern if a dog is bringing a client a toy to play with because the dog is merely bored and wants to play or because the dog is trying to lighten the distressed mood of the client. Much of the time one can only guess at what an animal is conveying, but the more familiar a facilitator is with the animal, the more often the animal's behavior will be accurately comprehended in a session. So, the more a facilitator works in partnership with a particular animal, the better the discernment of what the animal is signaling in relation to the client in a session will be. Also, it might be possible to discern what the animal may be signaling by simply asking the client what they believe the animal is communicating in relation to what the client is feeling or thinking at that moment. Regardless of whether the client's speculation about the animal is accurate, something of value is usually revealed about the client. Because therapy animals are relational beings, human clients may tend to project onto the animal's behavior a meaning that arises from the client's own imaginings formulated by way of the client's inner experiences. These projections by the client can represent conscious and unconscious motivational forces of the client (e.g., needs, wants, desires).

Animals that are mammals should not be considered objects. Instead, they must be considered social beings, and this is their greatest contribution to animal-assisted psychotherapy—that is, their socialness. The greatest asset of animals in psychotherapy sessions is their relational value. An AAT facilitator must recognize the social-relational value of HAI and work from the perspective of significant human-animal relational moments to move a client more effectively toward the desired goals (Chandler 2018).

Animal-Assisted Interventions in Psychotherapy

A therapeutic intervention can be divided into two parts: the technique used by a therapist and the intention for using the technique. The intention is the purpose or reason for using the technique, otherwise stated as what a therapist hopes to accomplish by facilitating a technique. O'Callaghan (2008, pp. 54, 104–105) conducted a comprehensive review of literature related to AAT applications in mental health and identified 18 techniques and 10 intentions or purposes for using AAT techniques. The 18 AAT techniques identified include the following:

1. Therapist reflects or comments on client's relationship with therapy animal.
2. Therapist encourages client to interact with therapy animal by touching or petting therapy animal.
3. Therapist encourages client to play with therapy animal during session.
4. Therapist encourages client to tell therapy animal about client's distress or concerns.
5. Therapist and client engage with therapy animal outside of a traditional therapeutic environment (i.e., taking therapy animal for a walk).
6. Therapist interacts with therapy animal by having animal perform tricks or follow commands.
7. Therapist encourages client to perform tricks with therapy animal.
8. Therapist encourages client to perform commands with therapy animal.
9. Therapist comments or reflects on spontaneous client-animal interactions.
10. Information about therapy animal's family history (e.g., lineage, breed, species) is shared with client.
11. Other history related to therapy animal is shared with client.
12. Animal stories and metaphors with animal themes are shared with client by therapist.
13. Therapist encourages client to make up stories involving therapy animal.
14. Therapist uses client–therapy animal relationship, such as "If this dog were your best friend, what would he know about you that no

one else would know?" or "Tell Rusty [therapy dog] how you feel, and I will just listen."

15. Therapist encourages client to re-create/reenact an experience where therapy animal plays a specific role.
16. Therapy animal is present without any directive interventions.
17. Therapist creates specific structured activities for client with therapy animal.
18. Therapy animal engages with client in spontaneous moments that facilitate therapeutic discussion.

The 10 AAT intentions identified were

A. Building rapport in the therapeutic relationship
B. Facilitating insight
C. Enhancing client's social skills
D. Enhancing client's relationship skills
E. Enhancing client's self-confidence
F. Modeling a specific behavior
G. Encouraging sharing of feelings
H. Creating a behavioral reward for client
I. Enhancing trust within the therapeutic environment
J. Facilitating feelings of being safe in the therapeutic environment

These lists of 18 AAT techniques and 10 AAT intentions are referred to by corresponding numbers and letters in other parts of the chapter.

The 18 techniques and 10 intentions identified from the literature review by O'Callaghan (2008) were used to develop a survey that was then distributed to 31 mental health therapists who practiced AAT to determine whether and how often therapists used these techniques and with what intentions (O'Callaghan and Chandler 2011). The results of the survey showed that although all of the techniques were used by most therapists, some techniques were used more often by a majority of the therapists; these were techniques 1, 2, 9, 16, and 18 (from the previous list of AAT techniques). The survey results also showed that AAT techniques were applied for a variety of intentions, but some intentions were clearly more common than others; for instance, one of the most common intentions for the use of techniques 1, 2, 10, and 11 was intention A, that of building rapport in the therapeutic relationship (O'Callaghan and Chandler 2011).

Researchers used information provided in the literature review by O'Callaghan (2008) to propose ways in which AAT could be applied within the parameters of a variety of psychotherapy guiding theories, including person-centered, cognitive-behavioral, Adlerian, psycho-analytic, gestalt, existential, reality/choice, and solution-focused, as described later in this chapter (Chandler et al. 2010). In their work, the researchers paired various intentions and techniques with specific theories based on obvious construct consistency; however, the researchers cautioned against any implication that some intentions and techniques were suited only for certain theories. They concluded that the versatility of AAT applications most likely makes this practice useful from the perspective of any psychotherapy guiding theory (Chandler et al. 2010), as is summarized in the following subsections.

Person-Centered Approach

When a person-centered approach (Tudor and Worrall 2006) is considered, some AAT techniques thought to be consistent with person-centered psychotherapy (Chandler et al. 2010) include reflecting on the client's relationship with the therapy animal (1), reflecting on spontaneous client–therapy animal interactions (9), having a therapy animal be present without any directive interventions (16), and having a therapeutic discussion of spontaneous interactions between the client and the therapy animal (18). Some AAT intentions thought to be consistent with a person-centered approach to psychotherapy include building rapport in the therapeutic relationship (A) and enhancing trust within the therapeutic environment (I), which enhances clients' sense of safety (J) and thereby encourages them to share their feelings (G), which may facilitate client insight (B) and, in turn, foster client self-acceptance or self-confidence (E) (Chandler et al. 2010).

Cognitive-Behavioral Approach

Many animal-assisted techniques and intentions are thought to be well suited for cognitive-behavioral therapy (Chandler et al. 2010; McMullin 1986). The therapist can use the client–therapy animal relationship to assist a client in expressing feelings or identifying beliefs (14). Clients can be guided to practice certain social skills with a therapy animal (15). The therapist can model appropriate social behaviors with a therapy animal (6). The therapist can ask a client to practice new and more functional behaviors with a therapy animal when engaging the animal to perform tricks or commands (7, 8). Similarly, the therapy animal can be involved in structured activities (17) to assist a client in learning and practicing new skills. Practicing new, positive behaviors with an animal first may be much more fun and much less threatening than trying them out on other humans. The use of appropriate humor by a therapist is an aspect of cognitive-behavioral psychotherapy and can be assisted through encouragement to play with an animal during a session (3). A therapist's feedback on all client–therapy animal interactions (1, 9) can assist a client in identifying functional and dysfunctional behaviors and reinforce client adaptation to more prosocial behaviors. Each of the following AAT intentions is thought to be consistent with the goals of cognitive-behavioral psychotherapy: building rapport (A) and enhancing trust (I) in the therapeutic relationship; encouraging sharing of feelings (G); gaining insight (B) about the consequences of feelings, thoughts, and actions; developing social and relationship skills (C, D); modeling specific behaviors (F); and enhancing the client's self-confidence (E) through successful interactions (Chandler et al. 2010).

Adlerian Approach

In the context of Adlerian psychotherapy (Carlson et al. 2006), several AAT intentions and techniques can be applied (Chandler et al. 2010). To establish an egalitarian therapeutic alliance as in Adlerian psychotherapy, a therapist can use AAT to facilitate rapport (A), trust (I), and feelings of safety (J) in a client. Adlerian therapists may use opportunities for social interaction among the client, therapist, and therapy animal to facilitate insight (B), to enhance the client's social and relationship skills (C, D), and to encourage the sharing of feelings (G). The Adlerian emphasis on social connectedness is consistent with nearly all AAT techniques. For example, all techniques involving interaction with a therapy animal are social in nature (1–9, 14–18). The Adlerian technique of gathering information on a client's family history can be facilitated by the therapist first sharing information about the therapy animal's family history (lineage, breed, or species) (10) as well as other personal history related to the therapy animal (11) (Chandler et al. 2010).

Psychoanalytic Approach

A psychoanalytic therapeutic approach (Hall 1954; Singer 1973) is thought to be compatible with AAT (Chandler et al. 2010) given that psychoanalytic therapists' primary role is to use the dynamics of the therapeutic relationship to facilitate client insight (B) and encourage the client to share their feelings (G). Therapists may do this by reflecting on the client's relationship with the therapy animal (1), reflecting on spontaneous client-animal interactions (9), and reflecting on how the animal engages with the client in spontaneous moments (18). The therapist can ask a client to make up stories about the therapy animal (13), allowing opportunity for the client to share unconscious thoughts and feelings by projecting them into the story. Animal stories and metaphors with animal themes may be shared with a client by a therapist (12) to access unconscious processes that are well defended by the client (Chandler et al. 2010).

Gestalt Approach

Gestalt theory (Perls et al. 1980) and AAT are believed to be a good match in several ways (Chandler et al. 2010). AAT applications can assist with facilitation of sensory awareness and self-discovery in clients, in that clients having difficulty attaching words to internal states may be better able to process their bodily sensations and feelings when petting and interacting with a therapy animal (2, 18, G). Therapist-facilitated activities for a client involving a therapy animal (17) may help a client to become more aware of verbal and body language patterns, which may assist client insight (B) regarding life areas where the client has become stuck. Furthermore, clients who have difficulty expressing personal challenges and unfinished business may find it easier to first share their distress or concerns with the therapy animal in the presence of the therapist (4). Finally, therapists may assist clients in accessing internal conflicts by requesting that they make up stories involving the therapy animal (13) (Chandler et al. 2010).

Existential Approach

The basic tenets of an existential approach to psychotherapy (Cooper 2003) are thought to match well with AAT intentions and techniques (Chandler et al. 2010). The existential goals of enhancing self-awareness and searching for meaning are consistent with the AAT intention of facilitating insight (B). Clients' movement toward greater personal freedom and responsibility is achieved by letting go of hindrances resulting from feelings of guilt and anxiety; this can be facilitated by the AAT intention of encouraging sharing of feelings (G). Achieving greater personal freedom and responsibility contributes to the AAT intention of enhanced client self-confidence (E). The existential proposition of striving for identity and relationship with others is consistent with the AAT intentions of enhancing clients' social and relationship skills (C, D). By allowing spontaneous interactions to occur between the client and the therapy animal (18) and commenting on the nature of these interactions (1), therapists may help clients to become aware of fears or feelings that impair authentic living. Animal stories and metaphors with animal themes may be shared with a client by a therapist (12) as examples of authentic or inauthentic living (Chandler et al. 2010).

Reality Therapy and Choice Theory Approach

From the perspective of reality therapy and choice theory (Glasser 1999), several AAT intentions and techniques may facilitate progress (Chandler et al. 2010). HAIs can assist with the formation and maintenance of the all-important therapeutic alliance between the therapist and the client (A). Clients' motivation to attend and participate in psychotherapy may be supported by their desire to spend time with the therapy animal for reasons that range from having fun in HAIs (2, 3, 7, 8) to appreciating the animal's role in easing self-evaluation and change, such as by facilitating insight (B), encouraging sharing of feelings (G), enhancing trust within the therapeutic environment (I), and facilitating feelings of being safe in the therapeutic environment (J). Interactions with the therapy animal may challenge clients in ways very similar to the challenges in their lives with people; however, these challenges can appear to be less threatening with animals than they are with people (C, D, 1, 9). Therapist-facilitated examinations of the consequences of actions, thoughts, feelings, and behaviors in HAIs (14, 15, 16, 17, 18) can help clients to learn lessons that can be applied with greater confidence (E) to relationships with people (Chandler et al. 2010).

Solution-Focused Approach

A solution-focused psychotherapy approach (Macdonald 2007) is believed to be compatible with various aspects of AAT (Chandler et al. 2010). Given that trust in the therapeutic relationship is a determining factor in the outcome of solution-focused psychotherapy, AAT intentions and techniques that foster a therapeutic relationship can be very valuable, including building rapport in the therapeutic relationship (A), enhancing trust within the therapeutic environment (I), and facilitating feelings of being safe in the therapeutic environment (J). With solution-focused psychotherapy, the emphasis is on here-and-now situations rather than on the past, and client–therapy animal interactions can enhance clients' focus, attention, concentration, and skill-building (1, 7, 8,

9, 18). Additionally, solution-focused psychotherapy emphasizes the importance of finding solutions to problems, and interactions with therapy animals provide opportunities to learn and practice new social and relationship skills (15, 17, C, D, F) that can result in enhanced client self-confidence (E) (Chandler et al. 2010).

Recommendations

Any psychotherapist who wishes to practice AAT should have sufficient knowledge, skill competency, and the proper attitude (Stewart et al. 2016). Knowledge includes in-depth training and supervision in AAT practice, learning about animals and their behavior, and gaining an understanding of the ethical and respectful practice of AAT with regard to both humans and animals. A practitioner should have proficiency in psychotherapy skills as well as competency in the skills involved in applying AAT interventions. A therapist's attitude should focus on advocacy for the safety and welfare of both human clients and therapy animals. AAT is not so simple as just bringing a pet to work and seeing what happens. AAT is a complex, advanced form of psychotherapy practice, and safety and advocacy issues must be considered for both the animal and the client.

Resources

A list of recommended resources for the practice of AAT in psychotherapy is provided below.

Cynthia K. Chandler	*Animal-Assisted Therapy in Counseling,* 3rd Edition (2017)
Aubrey H. Fine (ed.)	*Handbook on Animal-Assisted Therapy: Foundations and Guidelines for Animal Assisted Interventions,* 5th Edition (2019)
Leif Hallberg	*The Clinical Practice of Equine-Assisted Therapy: Including Horses in Human Healthcare* (2017)
Kay Sudekum Trotter and Jennifer N. Baggerly (eds.)	*Equine-Assisted Mental Health for Healing Trauma* (2018)

References

Bachi K, Terkel J, Teichman M: Equine-facilitated psychotherapy for at-risk adolescents: the influence on self-image, self-control and trust. Clin Child Psychol Psychiatry 17(2):298–312, 2012 21757481

Carlson J, Watts R, Maniacci M: Adlerian Therapy: Theory and Practice. Washington, DC, American Psychological Association, 2006

Chandler CK: Animal-Assisted Therapy in Counseling, 3rd Edition. New York, Routledge, 2017, pp 103–140

Chandler CK: Human-animal relational theory: a guide for animal-assisted counseling. J Creat Ment Health 13(4):429–444, 2018

Chandler CK, Portrie-Bethke TL, Barrio Minton CA, et al: Matching animal-assisted therapy techniques and intentions with counseling guiding theories. J Ment Health Couns 32(4):354–374, 2010

Cooper M: Existential Therapies. Thousand Oaks, CA, Sage, 2003

Daley Olmert M: Made for Each Other: The Biology of the Human–Animal Bond. Philadelphia, PA, Da Capo Press, 2009

Dietz TJ, Davis D, Pennings J: Evaluating animal-assisted therapy in group treatment for child sexual abuse. J Child Sex Abuse 21(6):665–683, 2012 23194140

Filiatre JC, Millot JL, Eckerlin A: Behavioural variability of olfactory exploration of the pet dog in relation to human adults. Appl Anim Behav Sci 30(3–4):341–350, 1991

Glasser W: Choice Theory: A New Psychology of Personal Freedom. New York, Harper Perennial, 1999

Hall C: A Primer of Freudian Psychology. New York, World Publishing, 1954

Handlin L, Hydbring-Sandberg E, Nilsson A, et al: Short-term interaction between dogs and their owners: effects on oxytocin, cortisol, insulin and heart rate—an exploratory study. Anthrozoos 24(3):301–315, 2011

Macdonald A: Solution-Focused Therapy: Theory, Research and Practice. Los Angeles, CA, Sage, 2007

McMullin R: Handbook of Cognitive Therapy Techniques. New York, WW Norton, 1986

O'Callaghan DM: Exploratory study of animal assisted therapy interventions used by mental health professionals. Doctoral dissertation, University of North Texas, May 2008. Available at: https://digital.library.unt.edu/ark:/67531/metadc6068/. Accessed February 5, 2022.

O'Callaghan DM, Chandler CK: An exploratory study of animal-assisted interventions utilized by mental health professionals. J Creat Ment Health 6(2):90–104, 2011

Odendaal JS: Animal-assisted therapy: magic or medicine? J Psychosom Res 49(4):275–280, 2000 11119784

Odendaal JS, Meintjes RA: Neurophysiological correlates of affiliative behaviour between humans and dogs. Vet J 165(3):296–301, 2003 12672376

Panksepp J: Affective Neuroscience: The Foundations of Human and Animal Emotions. New York, Oxford University Press, 2004

Panksepp J: Affective consciousness: core emotional feelings in animals and humans. Conscious Cogn 14(1):30–80, 2005 15766890

Perls F, Hefferline R, Goodman P: Gestalt Therapy. New York, Bantam, 1980

Prothmann A, Bienert M, Ettrich C: Dogs in child psychotherapy: effects on state of mind. Anthrozoos 19(3):265–277, 2006

Rørvang MV, Nielsen BL, McLean AN: Sensory abilities of horses and their importance for equitation science. Front Vet Sci 7:633, 2020 33033724

Rugaas T: Calming Signals: What Your Dog Tells You. Wenatchee, WA, Dogwise Publishing, 2005

Singer J: Boundaries of the Soul: The Practice of Jung's Psychology. Garden City, NY, Anchor, 1973

Singletary M, Lazarowski L: Canine special senses: considerations in olfaction, vision, and audition. Vet Clin North Am Small Anim Pract 51(4):839–858, 2021 34059259

Stewart LA, Chang CY, Parker LK, Grubbs N: Animal-Assisted Therapy in Counseling Competencies. Alexandria, VA, American Counseling Association, Animal-Assisted Therapy in Mental Health Interest Network, 2016. Available at: https://www.counseling.org/docs/default-source/competencies/animal-assisted-therapy-competencies-june-2016.pdf?sfvrsn=14. Accessed March 17, 2022.

Trotter KS, Chandler CK, Goodwin-Bond D, Casey J: A comparative study of the efficacy of group equine assisted counseling with at-risk children and adolescents. J Creat Ment Health 3(3):254–284, 2008

Tudor K, Worrall M: Person-Centered Therapy: A Clinical Philosophy. New York, Routledge, 2006

Uvänas-Moberg K, Arn I, Magnusson D: The psychobiology of emotion: the role of the oxytocinergic system. Int J Behav Med 12(2):59–65, 2005 15901214

17

Take-Home Messages

Nancy R. Gee, Ph.D.
Lisa D. Townsend, Ph.D., LCSW
Robert L. Findling, M.D., M.B.A.

THE INTRODUCTION to this volume highlighted two important themes running throughout the chapters: 1) the potential for companion animals to participate in positive and impactful ways in the treatment of mental illnesses and 2) the importance of respecting all animals involved and finding ways to ensure their overall quality of life. Indeed, the heart of this book (Chapters 6–13) details the variety of ways that companion animals may be involved in the treatment of a range of mental illnesses and challenging circumstances. These chapters have shown that animals may participate effectively in the treatment of ADHD (Chapter 6) and autism spectrum disorder (Chapter 7), reduce depression (Chapter 8), decrease stress and anxiety (Chapter 9), and contribute to the treatment of PTSD (Chapter 10) and serious mental illness (Chapter 11). Furthermore, companion animals can be a positive addition to crisis intervention (Chapter 4) and palliative care settings (Chapter 12) and play a role in the treatment of dementia and aging-related concerns (Chapter 13) and at-risk and adjudicated youth (Chapter 5).

As can be seen in the individual chapters, the current goal in human-animal interaction (HAI) research and practice is to move the entire field to a higher level of awareness and implementation of animal welfare and well-being standards. Clinicians and researchers are encouraged to understand and to address the needs of the animals involved in animal-assisted activities, animal-assisted therapy (AAT), and animal-assisted interventions (AAIs). Chapter 2 inspires clinicians to better understand canine welfare issues, to recognize signs of stress in canines, to identify canine attributes that contribute to effective AAT and AAIs, and to appropriately select dogs for work in AAT, AAIs, and animal-assisted activities. Importantly, this chapter discusses the therapeutic alliance, notes contraindications for animal involvement in clinical settings, and highlights the role of the clinician in identifying and intervening in animal abuse situations. Chapter 3 discusses clinician competencies, including animal welfare and well-being considerations and the effect of pets on mental health, and describes and distinguishes among the distinct roles that dogs play in mental health care and treatment.

Finally, Chapters 14–16 provide specific examples of and guidance about how our animal partners can serve as effective adjuncts to treatment: Chapter 14 describes the incorporation of AAIs in a university setting; Chapter 15 showcases a model dog visitation program that has been shown to provide a variety of benefits in a hospital setting; and Chapter 16 provides a broad overview of how AAT can be incorporated into the delivery of psychotherapy in a variety of settings and with an array of different patient populations.

Each chapter in this volume summarizes the current state of the science within each topical area, and several themes emerge from these summaries. First, evidence suggests that companion animals can be an effective adjunct to the treatment of mental illness. It is not suggested that companion animals may replace accepted treatment approaches (e.g., medications and psychotherapy); rather, it is pointed out that animals can participate in a way that reduces symptoms and/or enhances the therapeutic context.

What Don't We Know?

A common refrain in conclusion sections of published HAI research is that more research is needed, specifically research meeting higher-quality standards. Although the field is making great strides, many gaps remain in the literature. For example, we need a better understanding of the animal side of the equation. What species (e.g., dogs, cats, horses) are most effective, and what aspects of the interaction (e.g., touching, watching) with the animal are critical to the accrual of any benefits? The field needs to establish some general guidelines for dosage in specific settings. Can the intervention be delivered in groups, or is individual animal interaction required? How many interactions are required, and how long must each individual interaction last? We are getting partial answers to some of these questions, but the accumulation of many individual studies and larger multisite randomized clinical trials will help us to genuinely fill in these important gaps in our understanding, so that we can most effectively deploy our limited animal resources to those participants and contexts that are most likely to benefit.

Related to this important topic of deploying resources efficiently is the corollary that we do not want to put animals into situations that have the potential to be stressful to them, particularly if the possible benefit to patients of doing so is small or nonexistent. The science on HAI rarely includes individuals who do not already have an affinity for animals, or who may be allergic to animals. Thus, we do not know whether individuals in these groups may benefit from interacting with companion animals. As much as the field of HAI needs to determine when animals may be a beneficial adjunct to treatment, we also must clearly delineate those situations in which animals are not beneficial and make available a set of clear recommendations for mental health professionals.

Furthermore, we must consider cultural and diversity issues related to accessing companion animals and AAIs and AATs. Based on the information presented in Chapter 1, there is reason to believe that companion animals may be particularly beneficial to marginalized groups, but access to these animals also may be more difficult for people with fewer resources. As we saw in Chapter 13, older adults benefit from companion animals in several ways, but when these individuals move into long-term care facilities, they are often required to give up their pets. This causes them much distress and makes the transition to the new facility more traumatic. Researchers, practitioners, and members of the general public need to recognize the importance and the effect of companion animals on the lives of so many diverse and potentially vulnerable groups and find ways to support companion animal ownership or interaction, because doing so supports the principles of diversity, equity, and inclusion.

Do People Need to Own a Pet to Benefit?

The research summarized in this volume clearly indicates that the strongest evidence for the health-related benefits of animals comes from studies involving animal interaction (e.g., AAIs, AAT, animal-assisted activities) rather than pet ownership. This suggests that it is not necessary to own a pet to benefit from companion animals. Pet ownership requires a time and financial commitment that may not be reasonable for some individuals on the basis of their current life circumstances. That does not mean, however, that they cannot benefit from interacting with pets. In fact, this idea is also extremely popular—Google displayed 4.69 billion hits on the phrase "How can I interact with dogs without owning one?" (search conducted March 20, 2022).

Mental health providers are encouraged to explore some of those suggestions on behalf of their clients, but if they are looking for something more clearly linked as an adjunct to ongoing treatment, then we suggest exploring local resources for animal-assisted activities, AAIs, and AAT. The American Kennel Club provides a listing of all therapy dog organizations (www.akc.org/sports/title-recognition-program/therapy-dog-program/therapy-dog-organizations). It is important to keep in mind, however, that program requirements, including behavior and health evaluations, for both humans and animals vary widely across these programs. If a mental health provider is interested in incorporating AAT into their own clinical practice, we recommend pursuing training specific to their therapeutic approach and setting. Several certificate programs are available that focus on training professionals to practice AAT ethically and humanely, and we encourage practitioners to do their due diligence in finding a reputable program that is well suited to their specific goals.

Who Is Likely to Benefit?

When considering the inclusion of AAIs, AAT, or animal-assisted activities as an adjunct to ongoing treatment, or even as a way to enhance overall well-being, it is important to consider who is most likely to benefit from interacting with, or owning, a companion animal. Likewise, we must be aware of those individuals for whom animal interaction is not recommended or may be risky because of concerns about neglect, violent or abusive behavior, or severe allergic reaction. This topic has been discussed throughout the volume, so we will not detail the issues here. Instead, we provide a simple take-home message: pets are not a panacea. Not everyone likes animals. Some people are allergic to animals. Some people have violent outbursts that can put an animal at risk, whereas others may not have the capacity to attend to the needs of an animal, putting that animal at risk for neglect. Some people have religious or cultural traditions that discourage them from interacting with animals. In short, practitioners must carefully evaluate each client's individual needs and situation before suggesting AAIs, AAT, or animal-assisted activities as an adjunct.

What Does the Future Hold?

There is a good argument for taking a One Health approach to the involvement of animals in the treatment of mental illness and as potential catalysts for mental health. At the core of One Health is the idea that we are all interconnected (Zinsstag et al. 2018). The One Health model puts forth the idea that the health of humans, animals (i.e., nonhuman animals), and the environment should be evaluated in unison such that the well-being of all three is considered (Carver 2020). Traditionally, the One Health model has treated animals as vectors for disease, but recent research in the field of HAI has initiated a new approach to One Health that extends its application to human and animal mental health and well-being. Examples of this idea include programs designed to support human health that can also include supports for companion animals. To illustrate, there are programs in place that provide transportation for qualified older adults to get to and from their medical appointments. Similar transportation services could help those same older adults to transport their companion animals to and from their veterinary appointments. Likewise, animal-related programs could potentially include elements that also support human health and well-being. For example, veterinary offices could link pet owners to pet-walking groups or pet-loss support services. A One Health approach considers the needs of animals in addition to those of humans. For example, older adults often report increased loneliness and social isolation, while many animals are placed in shelters and need interaction and training in preparation for adoption. Pairing these two groups by actively recruiting older adults as animal shelter volunteers can improve the health and well-being of both (Carver 2020).

We have seen in this volume that the popular notion of companion animals as beneficial to the health and well-being of humans is partially supported by science, but we must be careful not to overgeneralize or romanticize those benefits. We are moving into a new era of understanding that the benefits of interacting with animals are real and can be profound, but we also need to manage our expectations about what animals can and cannot do. To accomplish this, we need to have a clear understanding of the needs of our animal partners, we need to respect them as valuable to the process, and we need to grant them agency to decline to participate.

Research efforts in the field of complementary and integrative medicine are beginning to consider holistic health and mental health, meaning that there is more to being well than the absence of illness. This mindset is consistent with the One Health approach in that determinants of health and well-being are found not only in individual biology but also in behavior, social relationships, and the wider environmental context. A holistic health focus also considers how nontraditional treatments such as AAIs can be woven into standard care.

Funding in support of rigorous scientific evaluation of complementary treatments for general medical and mental health conditions continues to grow. This book has provided an overview of the state of HAI science with respect to mental health and, it is hoped, given the reader a sense of how far the field has come since animals first became involved in formal mental health services. As HAI science advances toward an understanding of the emotional and biological mechanisms mutually invoked during HAIs, we will develop a greater ability to tailor animal-assisted activities, AAIs, and AAT to better match patients and animals for the mutual benefit of each. We look forward to deepening our understanding of how, why, and for whom animals bring much-needed relief from the emotional pain of mental illness and how we can harness scientific knowledge to improve the lives of both people who have psychiatric symptoms and the animals who share our lives, our feelings, and our planet.

References

Carver LF: One Health: fostering hope for older adults and homeless companion animals. People Anim 3(1):2, 2020

Zinsstag J, Crump L, Schelling E, et al: Climate change and One Health. FEMS Microbiol Lett 365(11):fny085, 2018 29790983

Index

Page numbers printed in **boldface** type refer to tables and figures.